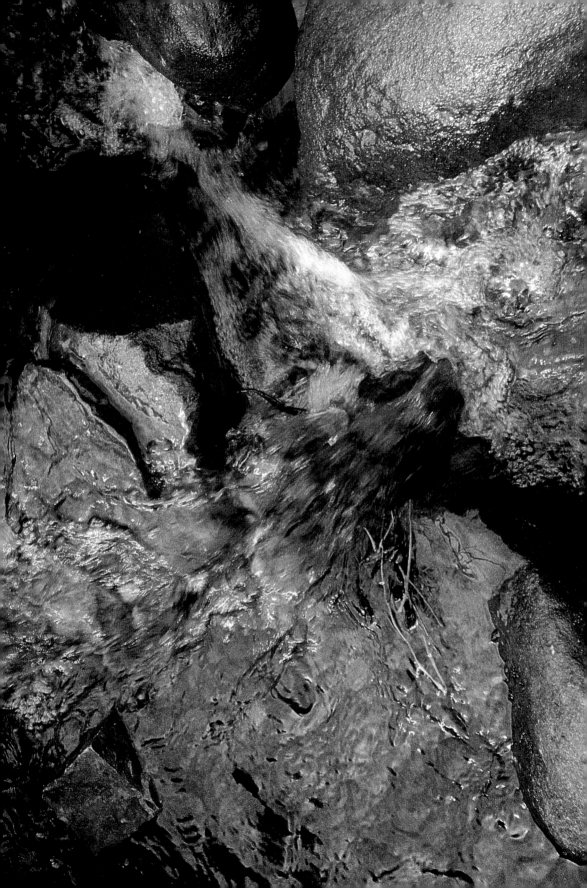

AROMATHERAPY
For HEALING THE SPIRIT

*A guide to restoring emotional and mental
balance through essential oils*

GABRIEL MOJAY

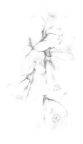

An Owl Book

Henry Holt and Company

New York

Henry Holt and Company, Inc.
Publishers since 1866
115 West 18th Street
New York, New York 10011

Henry Holt® is a registered
trademark of Henry Holt and Company, Inc.

First published in the United States in 1996 by
Henry Holt and Company, Inc.
Published in Canada by Fitzhenry & Whiteside Ltd.,
195 Allstate Parkway, Markham, Ontario L3R 4T8.

Originally published in United Kingdom in 1996
by Gaia Books Ltd.

Library of Congress Cataloging-in-Publication Data

Mojay, Gabriel.
    Aromatherapy for healing the spirit : a guide to restoring
emotional and mental balance through essential oils / Gabriel Mojay.
        p.   cm.
    "An Owl book."
    Includes bibliographical references and index.
    I. Aromatherapy.   I. Title.
    RM666.A68M65 1996
    615'.321--dc20   95-49041
                                                              CIP

ISBN 0-8050-4496-5

Henry Holt books are available for special promotions and
premiums. For details contact: Director, Special Markets.

First American Edition—1996

Editor	Joanna Godfrey Wood
Designers	Phil Gamble and Sara Mathews
Illustrator	Johanna Amos
Managing Editor	Pip Morgan
Production	Susan Walby
Direction	Patrick Nugent

Printed in Singapore
All first editions are printed on acid-free paper ∞

10 9 8 7 6 5 4 3 2 1

For Chester and Caz

TO THE READER
The psychological and therapeutic benefits of the
essential oils discussed in this book are based on
traditional knowledge and experience. The context of their use as presented in the text is that of
complementary health care – of the individual,
the family, and the fee-paying client, for
purposes of both self-help and professional aromatherapy. The concepts, suggestions, and
techniques outlined herein are not intended as a
substitute for medical advice. Any application of
the ideas and information contained in the book
is at the reader's sole discretion and risk.

CAUTION
*Essential oils should never be taken by mouth unless
prescribed by a medical doctor, or a qualified practitioner who has trained to a medical standard.
Essential oils should only be applied to the skin
diluted in a carrier oil, cream, or gel.*

Contents

Part One

Part Two

Part Three

Appendix

Foreword

by Robert Tisserand

Western medical doctors were thrown into a state of utter confusion when first presented with anaesthesia by acupuncture in the early 1970s. Some travelled to China to witness at first hand the most traumatic of medical procedures – heart surgery – being performed with acupuncture needles as the only form of pain control. Fascinated and perplexed, they urgently sought a rational, scientific explanation for something which appeared impossible.

The mind boggles when presented with evidence of highly sophisticated ancient knowledge. Like the pyramids of Egypt, traditional Chinese medicine is a massive edifice – one which is built, not of stone but of painstaking observation, practice, and skill. It is a body of wisdom that has accumulated over the millennia through the work of thousands of practitioners.

Making this inherently complex subject accessible and real, and at the same time merging it with the practice of aromatherapy, is no easy task, but one which Gabriel Mojay accomplishes with clarity and confidence. The text is dense with insight, and yet concise and easy to reference. Every page draws the reader inexorably into an intricate web of holistic truth.

The main focus is on the psychological energetic plane, although in this truly holistic approach, mind and body cannot really be separated. The reader will find a complete rationale for selecting essential oils appropriate to the needs of the whole person, and many aromatherapists will find this ancient yet novel approach an enlightening one. This is the first useful text on the energetics of essential oils, and it helps to give authority and substance to an area inherently esoteric and diffuse.

In combining the practice of aromatherapy with the wisdom of Oriental medicine, Gabriel has certainly given a new dimension to aromatherapy. He may also have added a little to Oriental medicine. For thousands of years, needles and herbs were the two principal avenues of treatment in China, and, to a large extent, still are. With essential oils, a third avenue opens up.

Introduction
the medicine of the Spirit

It is often said that the source of most illness has its roots in the depths of the soul. Indeed, it is a belief that was held even by Plato, and in traditional societies by the medicine man.

This is consistent with the fact that the people of such societies often make no distinction between spirit and matter. The "primitive" world view is commonly one of spiritual *immanence* – of the indwelling nature of the spiritual, and of its inseparable relationship to the material. It is an outlook that runs counter to the dualistic assumption that the body and mind are mutually separate. The body and its functions are seen instead as direct expression of a conscious, guiding principle.

Much of the wisdom of Oriental medicine lies in the appreciation of this very fact – that while "vital substances" such as *blood* and *body fluids* are manifestations of energy, energy itself – known as *Qi* (pronounced "chi") – is, like the conscious mind, yet another type of "substance".

This understanding is of value both to the practice of aromatherapy and the use of essential oils generally. For what better way to influence the mind and Spirit than through a physical medium that captures with such evocative power the very essence of Nature? Essential oils, too, are "vital substances" – the natural alchemical synergy of plant and sun.

The goal of this book, therefore, is to provide the necessary "tools" to perceive and apply the oils as messengers of energy and consciousness. By considering the botanical, traditional, and energetic aspects of each essential oil, we will be able to distill its psychological and spiritual "resonance", and the unique healing force that it yields.

As Oriental medicine affords us, in addition, an appreciation of the uniqueness of the *individual*, it is then simply a case of matching the person's needs with the vital properties of a particular oil or oils.

The book itself is divided into three parts: Part I will provide you with the therapeutic foundations to using essential oils from a psychological and basic perspective. You will then be able to comprehend fully the discussion of the oils in Part II, and apply them, in turn, to the restoring of balance addressed in Part III of the book. It is here that we shall seek to answer the call for the aromatic *medicine of the Spirit*.

"To reach the individual we need an individual remedy. Each of us is a unique message. It is only the unique remedy that will suffice. We must, therefore, seek odiferous substances which present affinities with the human being we intend to treat, those which will compensate for his deficiencies and those which will make his faculties blossom."

MARGUERITE MAURY
The Secret of Life and Youth

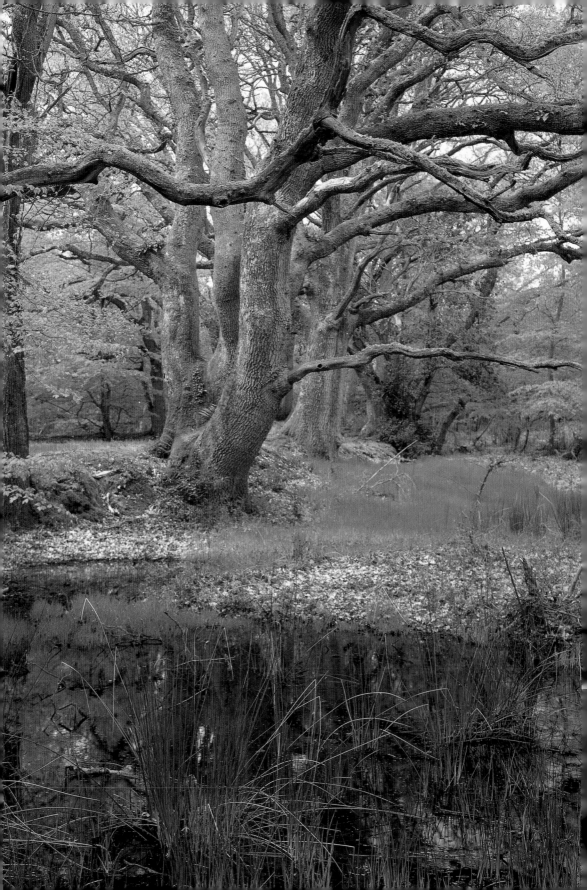

Part One
Therapeutic Foundations

THE POND REMINDS US OF THE TREE'S NEED FOR MOISTURE
"Water generates Wood"

Aromatic plants have been used by humankind since the dawn of history. There is evidence that over some 4,000 years ago, the Ancient Sumerians made use of scented herbs such as cypress and myrrh, while in the 1870s George Ebers discovered a 21-metre (70-foot) scroll of papyrus that listed over 850 Ancient Egyptian botanical remedies, dating from about 1500 BC.

That the Ancient Egyptians – or indeed the Greeks – were masters of the science of distillation is doubtful – yet it is certain that stills of a primitive kind were used to catch aromatic steam, and that this and other methods allowed them to produce both perfumes and ointments.

Practices such as these were the beginnings of a tradition that embraced not one but several civilizations, and developed hand-in-hand with systems of science and medicine that were based on both empirical knowledge and informed intuition.

Ancient Greek physicians such as Hippocrates and Galen interpreted the microcosm of the human being according to the Elements of Fire, Water, Earth, and Air, while the masters of the Chinese tradition saw Five Elements at work. In either case, they employed a rich and varied language of Nature – not to describe their observations as fixed phenomena, but like the physicists of today, to use these concepts to expose the dynamic force that masquerades as matter.

By applying traditional wisdom to aromatherapy, we can avail ourselves of a corpus of knowledge that is both immediate and profound, practical and intuitive. And through contributing to the synthesis of East and West, we can expand our awareness both of the human spirit and the plant essence.

Essential Oils & Aromatherapy

an overview

Aromatherapy can be defined as the controlled use of essential oils to maintain and promote physical, psychological, and spiritual wellbeing. Essential oils are volatile (easily evaporated) substances that occur naturally in a variety of plants growing the world over. Each plant essence is extracted from a single botanical source through a number of possible methods, the most common and generally favoured being that of steam distillation. Essential oils are highly aromatic, and are the main traditional constituents of most perfumes and fragrances. The scent of an oil makes a vital contribution to its natural healing properties.

Essential oils are synthesized and stored in many parts of the plant, and in several different types of secretory structures. Essential oils of eucalyptus and tea tree *(Myrtaceae* family), for example, occur in oil sacs *within* the leaf, while those of peppermint and clary sage *(Labiatae)* are found in glands *on* the leaf surface. Oil of rose *(Rosaceae)* is extracted from the petals of the flower, and clove oil *(Myrtaceae)*, from the dried flower buds. In the case of marjoram oil *(Labiatae)*, the flowering tops are used – including petals, sepals, upper stalks, and leaves – while to produce oil of yarrow *(Compositae)*, the entire herb is distilled. Juniper *(Cupressaceae)* yields an essence from both its berries and twigs, and orange *(Rutaceae)*, from its flowers, leaves, and the rind of its fruits. Plants that belong to the *Umbelliferae* family, including fennel, caraway, and coriander, bear their oil in the seeds, just as those of *Burseraceae* – such as frankincense and myrrh – occur in the bush's resin.

Essential oils produced from the chopped wood of trees include cedarwood *(Pinaceae)* and sandalwood *(Santalaceae)*, while those of pine and spruce *(Pinaceae)* are distilled mainly from the needles (or leaves). Vetiver *(Gramineae)* is an example of an oil extracted from the root, and ginger *(Zingiberaceae)*, from the fragrant rhizome. It is not completely understood *why* plants manufacture essential oils, but it is becoming clear that they fulfill some important ecological functions. There is evidence, for example, that the

ESSENTIAL OIL
This symbol is the medieval alchemical sign for essential oil. The quality of an essential oil's aroma is determined by the health of the plant from which it is derived. If properly distilled and handled, essential oils produced from wild or organically grown plants will always convey through their fragrance a sense of vitality and Qi (life force).

essences of some plants attract pollinating insects, while others serve a repellent function. And just as essential oils possess, on a therapeutic level, powerful antimicrobial properties, so in nature do they often display the potential to prevent attack by fungi and bacteria.

There are a number of methods by which the volatile components of aromatic plants may be extracted for commercial purposes. However, such a volatile product cannot be considered a true essential oil unless it has been produced either through distillation or cold expression. The process of steam distillation begins when the distiller inserts the chosen plant material, or *charge*, into a special chamber. Often at considerable pressure, steam is then forced into the chamber. As it passes through the plant material, the steam ruptures the plant's oil-bearing sacs and cavities, and liberates its essence, which consequently evaporates into the steam. The steam and vaporized essential oil then pass out of the chamber and through a coiled tube surrounded by cold water. Here, they

THE DISTILLATION PROCESS
This representation of a traditional still shows steam passing through plant material, carrying its volatile components out through the top of the chamber. The steam and vaporized essence then condense to form fragrant water (hydrolat) and essential oil. Because the oil collects on the water's surface, it is easily drained off and collected in a hand-held flask.

DISTILLATION CHAMBER

STEAM AND VAPOURIZED OIL

CONDENSING CHAMBER

COLD WATER INLET

PLANT MATERIAL

STEAM

WATER & ESSENTIAL OIL

BOILING WATER

ESSENTIAL OIL OUTLET

FRAGRANT WATER

FIRE

condense into water and liquid essential oil, and flow into a collecting vase. The essential oil is unable to mix with water and so forms a layer above it, making it easy to separate. Small quantities of odorous principles also remain in the water, forming a fragrant water, or *hydrolat*. The hydrolat is often used to form the new distillation steam, and becomes more concentrated in the process. Floral waters such as rose and chamomile have been important for skin care and fragrance ever since distillation was discovered in the 13th century.

Fragrance materials can also be extracted with the aid of solvents such as hexane. However, the resulting product, called an *absolute*, is not a pure essential oil, as it contains additional plant constituents. Absolutes are unsuitable for therapeutic purposes, due to the small amount of toxic residue they will invariably contain. Solvent extraction, or *separation*, is often used to extract the aromatic principles from plants with a very low yield of essence, such as neroli and rose. It is generally favoured by the perfume industry as it is more economical than the distillation process.

Cold expression is a process used for the extraction of essential oils from the rind of citrus fruits. The outer layer of the peel is ruptured through mechanical means and the essence, or zest, pressed out. Cold-pressed grades of orange, bergamot, mandarin, grapefruit, lemon, and lime oils are obtained in this way.

The traditional process of *enfleurage* is still occasionally used to extract the aromatic components of delicate flowers such as jasmine. A layer of fresh flowers is placed on a thin layer of odourless animal fat, called the *chassis*. The fat gradually becomes saturated with the aromatic constituents of the flower, and is then treated with alcohol to produce an *absolute ex pomade*. This process is very expensive and not widely used.

Distilled and expressed essential oils are composed of a wide variety of relatively simple compounds, made up in the main of carbon, hydrogen, and oxygen. These atoms, between them, combine to produce at least 3,000 different

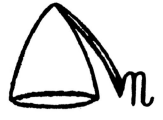

THE YIELD
This symbol is the medieval Alchemical sign for distillation. The proportion of essential oil that can be distilled from the plant material is called the "yield". This can range from 4 to 7% in the case of caraway seeds to as low as one- to four-tenths of a per cent in rose petals. It fact, it requires something like 60,000 roses to produce a single ounce (25g) of the essence!

aromatic molecules, each of which belongs to a specific chemical group, according to its basic structure.

Most essential oils are made up of molecules from several different chemical groups, though it is fairly common for just one or two groups to predominate. In the case of *Eucalyptus globulus*, for example, the major constituent is cineole, a compound that belongs to the oxide group. Although cineole constitutes up to 85% of the essential oil, other chemical groups are also represented. These include terpenes, alcohols, ketones, and aldehydes.

It is the unique combination of the plant's chemical constituents that determine both its synergy of therapeutic effects and its aroma. These cannot be imitated by a chemical mixture that is produced in the laboratory. It would be impossible to reproduce each of the numerous minute constituents that contribute to the aroma of a natural essential oil, nor conceivable that such a chemical cocktail would possess the life force of the authentic product.

The aroma of an essential oil and of fragrances generally is, according to perfumery, broken down into three basic components: "top", "middle", and "base" notes. An oil's *top notes* are those that are light and fresh in aroma, and the first that the nose will discern. They predominate in oils that evaporate more quickly, such as grapefruit and peppermint. The *middle notes* provide the heart, and often the bulk, of the fragrance, and are for this reason to be found in almost all essential oils. The *base notes* are heavy and rich in character, and are the last to emerge from the scent. They give to oils such as benzoin and patchouli a fixative capacity, as they evaporate slowly and have a strong tenacity. Essential oils, via the olfactory nerves, affect, among other parts of the brain, the limbic system – one of the most primitive regions of consciousness. Although they are the tools of a gentle therapy, essential oils have the power to reach deep into the psyche, and to both relax the mind and uplift the Spirit.

THE BURNER
Essential oil "burners" are becoming a popular way to fragrance the home. Place 5-20 drops of essential oil on some water in the shallow bowl that forms the top of the burner. Inside the burner, light a small candle to heat the water, so vaporizing the oil.

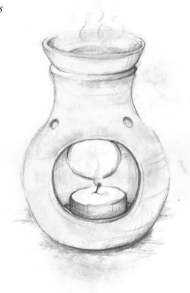

Methods of Application
how to use essential oils

There are various ways that one can apply essential oils – both for therapeutic benefit and pleasure. The following methods are the safest and most commonly used. They involve the skin absorption of essential oils through massage, ointments, compresses, and baths, as well as inhalation. Whichever method one chooses, their effect is always both physical and psychological.

Essential oils should never be taken by mouth unless prescribed either by a medical doctor, or a qualified practitioner who has trained to a medical standard (e.g. many medical herbalists).

The application of essential oils through aromatherapy massage is a method that is enhanced by the physiological benefits of massage itself. Its ability to promote the flow of blood and lymph and to improve nervous conductivity, give it the capacity both to soothe tension and increase vital energy. Safe and supportive, therapeutic touch also possesses the power to convey a sense of emotional wellbeing. Carried out by a well-trained practitioner, it can transform and renew.

During an aromatherapy massage, the aromatic molecules of the essential oils exert an influence both through their inhalation and smell, and through their cutaneous absorption. Although normally impermeable to water, the skin can absorb small, fat-soluble substances relatively easily. Once they pass through the skin's surface, they make their way to the dermis, the layer of the skin that is served by capillaries. It is here that the molecules enter general circulation.

The actual "dosage" of essential oil to be used is calculated as a percentage proportion of the carrier oil. This can vary from half to a maximum of three per cent, depending upon the individual and their condition. People with hypersensitive or allergic skin, those on orthodox drug medication, or women during pregnancy should receive only a half per cent dilution of essential oil. When utilizing essential oils for their psychological benefits, I would suggest a proportion of no more than one and a half per cent or three drops of essence for every 10ml (two standard teaspoons) of carrier oil.

For children, the amount of essential oil applied will be

THE CARRIER
Essential oils should never be applied to the skin "neat", and are always diluted in a carrier oil before they are used in massage. Among the many types of carrier oils available, professional aromatherapists will usually recommend cold-pressed vegetable oils such as almond, sunflower, and walnut.

reduced in proportion to the volume of carrier oil required to cover their smaller body surface. However, I would recommend that for children under 13, the proportion of essential oil should be reduced to one per cent or two drops of oil for every 10ml (two standard teaspoons) of carrier; and for children under three, that the proportion of essential oil should be reduced to half a per cent, or one drop of oil for every 10ml of carrier.

Aromatherapy massage should not be carried out on those with influenza or fever, or on someone who has just eaten a heavy meal, or taken alcohol. One should avoid massaging over recent scar tissue, skin infection, or extensive bruising. Do, not, in addition, massage around broken or fractured bones, and injured muscles or tendons. It is also better not to massage the legs in those with varicose veins, nor over areas where there is an inflammatory condition such as rheumatoid arthritis. In cases of heart disease, one should seek advice from a medical practitioner.

Aromatherapy massage is very beneficial during pregnancy, but avoid the abdominal area. It is also necessary to avoid using the following essential oils mentioned in the text: fennel, hyssop, peppermint, rosemary, and yarrow.

Aromatic ointments are made by adding essential oils to a cream or gel base. At a recommended proportion of two per cent of essential oil, add a total of 20 drops of essence to a 50g (2oz) jar. It is also recommended that you add five per cent (half a standard teaspoon) of cold-pressed wheatgerm oil to the ointment blend, as its vitamin E content contributes an antioxidant action which helps to prevent spoilage. In addition, the therapeutic properties of the ointment may be enhanced by adding between ten and twenty per cent (one to two teaspoons) of infused herbal oils such as those produced from marigold (*Calendula*

MAKING AN OINTMENT
Aromatic ointments are suitable for "local" application to a specific body area. They are made from a blend of essential oils, base cream or gel, wheatgerm oil, and optional infused herbal oils.

officinalis) and St John's Wort *(Hypericum perforatum).*

Compresses, like ointments, are an excellent way of applying essential oils to a specific area. *Hot* compresses are particularly beneficial for chronic backache, rheumatic pain, and osteoarthritis. To make a hot compress, fill a bowl with hot water. Add three to five drops of essential oil to the water. Place a folded piece of cotton cloth, cotton wool, or a flannel on to the water, wring out, and apply to the affected area. Repeat two to four times. A *cold* compress can be made in a similar way, but using cold water. It is useful for problems of an acute nature, including headaches, sprains, and bruises.

Steam inhalation helps to clear the lungs and sinus passages of mucous congestion and infection. Add two or three drops of essential oil to 6 litres (one pint) of boiled water. Draping a towel over the head, breathe in the steam for one or two minutes; then repeat. Discontinue if this causes discomfort.

One of the most pleasurable ways to utilize essential oils is through bathing – which both relaxes the nerves and soothes muscular aches and pains. For an adult add four to six drops of pure essential oil to very warm bath water, stirring it well. Relax in the bath for a good ten minutes.

There are numerous ways in which one can employ essential oils to fragrance a room, and take advantage of their ability to relax and clarify. Essential oil "burners" are now commonly available and involve the vaporization of oils from heated water. An alternative is to float a few drops of essential oil on a saucer of water near a warm radiator.

The most therapeutically effective means of dispersing essential oil into the air is through the use of an aromatic "nebulizer". Because the oil does not require heating, its chemical components remain unaltered, and is subsequently of greater benefit. Aerial dispersion decongests the air passages, enhances the breathing process and protects the body against air-borne viruses.

THE NEBULIZER

Nebulizers can be used to disperse essential oils into the air without the need to heat them. Under the power of an electric pump, a fine stream of air meets a stream of essential oil, and the oil is "vaporized" as a result.

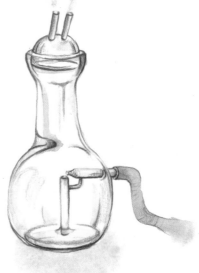

Methods of application

METHOD	PROCEDURE	DOSAGE	BENEFITS
Massage	*Use a massage couch and cover the person with towels, exposing areas one at a time. Massage for up to 90 minutes*	*7-10 drops (1.5- 2%) in 25ml (1fl oz) of carrier oil, for a complete massage (adult dose)*	*Benefits physical and psychological problems. Good for muscular fatigue and aching, nervous tension, and anxiety*
Ointments and creams	*These require a cream base, preferably made from cold-pressed vegetable oil. Apart from essential oil, one may add wheatgerm and herbal oils such as calendula and hypericum, at 10-20%*	*5-20 drops (0.5 -2%) in a 50g (2oz) jar or tub*	*Higher dose of 2% may be applied to bruises, sprains, painful joints, and the chest and back for respiratory ailments. Lower dose of 0.5% is for sensitive or inflamed skin*
Compress	*Add essential oil to a bowl of either hot or cold water. Place a cloth on the water and wring out. Apply to affected area for 5 mins. Repeat 2-4 times*	*3-5 drops in a 6-litre (one-pint) bowl of water*	*Hot compresses are suitable for cold conditions characterized by a fixed, cramping pain, worse in cold weather. Cold ones are for hot, swollen conditions, and pain of a "burning" nature*
Steam inhalation	*Add essential oil to a bowl of boiled water. Draping a towel over the head, breathe in the steam for 1-2 minutes only. Repeat 2-4 times*	*2-3 drops in a 6-litre (one-pint) bowl of water*	*Effective for respiratory complaints, including: bronchial and sinus congestion; coughs and bronchitis; and sore throats, colds, and influenza*
Bath	*Add essential oil to very warm bath water, vigorously stirring in the drops to ensure full and safe dispersal. Allow time for a good, relaxing soak*	*4-6 drops (adult) 3-5 drops (13-16 yrs) 2-4 drops (10-12 yrs) 1-3 drops (7-9 yrs) 1-2 drops (4-6 yrs) 1 drop (under 3 yrs)*	*The ultimate way to relax. Especially beneficial for nervous tension and tired, sore muscles. For insomnia, bathe in oils such as lavender, orange, and chamomile before going to bed*
Vaporization	*Add essential oil to a burner (containing water), or a dish of water that can be safely warmed. Or use an electric nebulizer (without water)*	*5-20 drops in a burner or dish; 20-200 drops in a nebulizer*	*A burner is best employed for the psychotherapeutic purposes of mood enhancement and upliftment. A nebulizer is preferable for disinfecting the air and to improve breathing*

Aromatherapy Massage
an introductory full-body sequence

EFFLEURAGE THE BACK OF THE LEG

Open your hands to separate thumbs from fingers, forming a "V" shape. Maintaining the "V", place your hands over the back of the ankle, and glide up the leg toward the thigh. At the thigh, separate your hands and let them gently glide back down the sides of the leg. Repeat, moving up and down in a continuous flow. Allow your hands to mould to the leg's contours. (Always use light pressure over the back of the knee.)

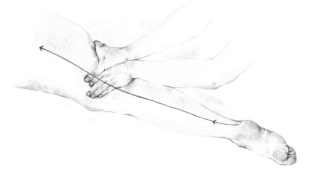

PETRISSAGE THE BACK OF THE LEG

Starting at the thigh, roll the thumb of one hand toward the fingers of the opposite hand. As thumb and fingers meet, the thigh muscles are lifted and gently squeezed. Continue this stroke using alternate thumb and fingers, moving from inner to outer thigh. Repeat this petrissage stroke on the calf, lifting and gently squeezing the calf muscle.

THUMB FRICTIONS UP EACH SIDE OF THE ACHILLES TENDON

Lift the leg at the ankle so that the foot is slightly raised. Using the balls of the thumbs, apply small circles of pressure on either side of the band of tendon that runs down the back of the ankle. Avoid making long sliding movements, as the thumb friction focuses on a small area just beneath the ball of the thumb. Work from the heel upward; then slide the thumbs down and repeat the stroke.

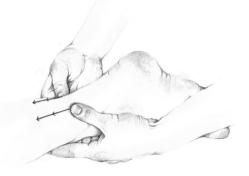

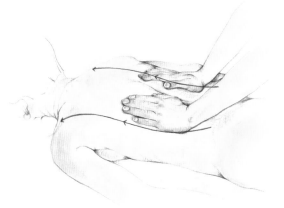

EFFLEURAGE THE BACK
Place your hands at the base of the back, either side of the spine. With fingertips pointing toward the shoulders, slowly glide your hands up the back. Move them across the top of the shoulders, then glide them down the sides of the body, returning to your starting point. Repeat, maintaining one continuous movement. A faster rhythm is more stimulating – a slower rhythm, more relaxing.

PETRISSAGE THE SHOULDER, SIDE OF BODY AND BUTTOCKS
Working on the opposite side of the body, start with your hands at the top of the shoulder, lifting and squeezing the muscles that lie across this area. Roll the thumb of one hand toward the fingers of the opposite hand; repeat using alternate thumb and fingers. Continue this movement down the side of the body to the buttocks. Repeat on the other side of the body.

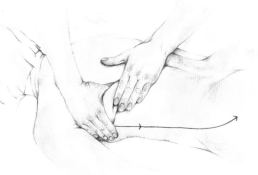

THUMB FRICTIONS UP THE BACK
Start with your thumbs at the base of the back, either side of the spine. Slowly work your way up the back, using the balls of your thumbs to make small circles of pressure. Each pressure, or "friction", focuses on a small area just beneath the ball of the thumb. At the shoulders, slide your hands down the back and repeat the stroke. (Be sure not to friction over the spine.)

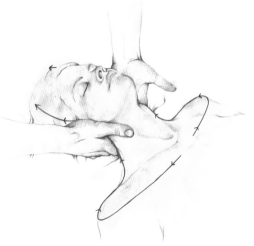

EFFLEURAGE THE NECK

Standing above the head, place your hands just above the breasts, with fingers facing each other. Slide your hands apart to the tip of the shoulders, then around and up the back of the shoulders toward the neck. Move them up the back of the neck, and behind the ears to the top of the head. Allow your hands to mould to the body's contours. (Avoid pressure on the front of the neck.)

FINGER FRICTIONS UP THE BACK OF THE NECK

Standing above the head, slide your fingers under the back of the neck, with fingertips facing each other. Starting at the base of the neck, use the balls of your middle three fingers to make small circles of pressure either side of the spine. Work slowly up the back of the neck and then along the base of the skull.

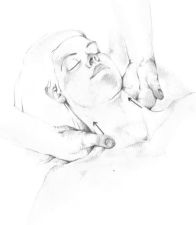

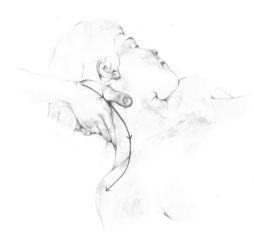

NECK STRETCH EFFLEURAGE

Hold the head in your hands, and gently rotate it to one side. Working on the side away from the face, place your palm, fingers pointing down, behind the ear; then slide your hand down the side of the neck and on to the tip of the shoulder. Keep the shoulder cupped in your palm and apply a gentle downward pressure to stretch the neck and shoulder. Repeat several times on each side. (Take care not to stretch beyond the limits of comfort.)

EFFLEURAGE THE CHEST

Standing on the side, place your palms on the midline of the chest, at the base of the rib cage. Slowly glide up the chest, between the breasts, and across the top of the shoulders. Glide your hands back down the sides of the body to the starting position. Repeat in one continuous stroke, allowing your hands to mould to the body's contours.

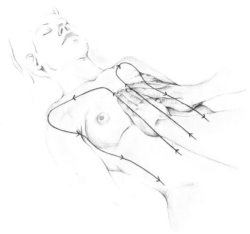

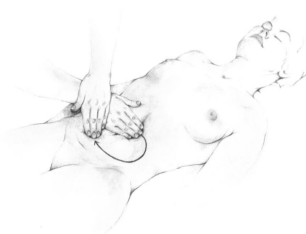

CIRCULAR EFFLEURAGE ON THE ABDOMEN

Standing on the side, imagine two semi-circles — one above and one below the navel. With your left hand lying flat on the abdomen, trace along both semi-circles in a clockwise direction. As your left hand moves away from you, place your right hand on the opposite side of the navel; let it semi-circle toward you, lifting it off the body to repeat. Maintain the stroke as one continuous movement.

DIAPHRAGMATIC RELEASE

This stroke helps to "release" the diaphragm muscle, which contributes to the breathing mechanism. Position your thumbs on the lower border of the rib cage, either side of the midline. Ask your partner to take a deep breath in. On the out-breath, slowly slide your thumbs outward, with palms and fingers resting gently on the body. Repeat. (Apply pressure only on the out-breath, to avoid constricting the breathing.)

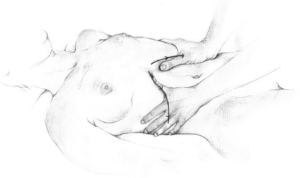

EFFLEURAGE THE ARM

This stroke uses alternate hands to glide up and down the arm in a smooth sequence. Holding your partner's hand slowly glide your other hand up the arm, around the shoulder, and back down the arm. Swap hands and repeat, maintaining one continuous movement. You can raise the arm to enable the gliding hand to reach the underside of the limb.

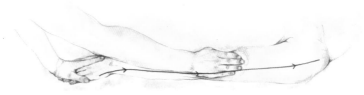

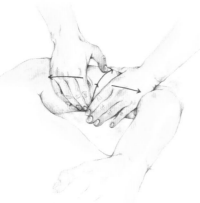

PETRISSAGE THE UPPER ARM

Bending your partner's elbow, bring their lower arm and hand to rest on the chest. Starting on the arm's inner surface, roll the thumb of one hand toward the fingers of the opposite hand. As thumb and fingers meet, the muscles of the inner arm are lifted and gently squeezed. Repeat using alternate thumb and fingers, moving from inner to outer arm.

THUMB EFFLEURAGE ON THE FOREARM

Hold the forearm at the wrist and gently raise it. Place the thumb of the free hand just above the wrist and slowly glide down the arm to the elbow. Draw your hand back up the arm to the wrist and repeat. Work your way around the forearm, working down to the elbow in parallel lines. While the focus is on thumb pressure, keep the rest of your hand in gentle contact with the arm.

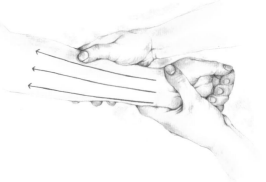

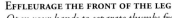

EFFLEURAGE THE FRONT OF THE LEG

Open your hands to separate thumbs from fingers, forming a "V" shape. Maintaining the "V", place your hands over the front of the ankle and glide up the centre of the leg toward the thigh. Separate your hands and let them glide back down the sides of the leg to the ankle. Repeat in a continuous rhythm, allowing your hands to mould to the contours of the leg. (Always use a very light pressure over the knee.)

WRINGING THE UPPER LEG

Placing your hands on either side of the thigh, bring the fingers of one hand toward the palm of the other, lifting and gently squeezing the large thigh muscle in between. Let your hands relax and return to the starting position to repeat. Use the lift-squeeze-and-relax cycle over the whole of the upper leg.

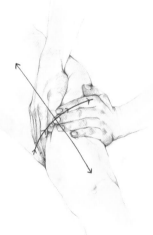

HEEL OF HAND EFFLEURAGE ON THE LOWER LEG

The "heel" of your hand is just below your wrist, and includes the fleshy pad below the thumb. Starting at the ankle, place the heel of both hands on either side of the shin bone and move them in a circular motion. Work up the sides of the shin to just below the knee; then slide your hands back to the starting position and repeat. Allow the thumb, fingers, and palm to maintain only gentle contact with the leg.

Yin & Yang

the foundations of Oriental medicine

The concept of *yin* and *yang* forms the basis of Oriental medicine. As a simple yet profound theory of *vital energy*, it can be applied to healing therapies of all kinds. Indeed, it constitutes the foundation of traditional approaches to herbal medicine, massage, diet, exercise and, of course, acupuncture.

The theory of *yin* and *yang* stretches back to the Chinese Zhou dynasty (1000-770 BC), when it appears in the *I-Ching*, or *Book of Changes*. Yet the fundamental polarity that *yin* and *yang* represents is not exclusive to Chinese medicine, and can be found at the root of the Western medical tradition as well.

Although the 2nd century Greek physician Galen makes no reference to the Chinese terms *yin* and *yang*, he nonetheless based his hugely influential herbal writings on strikingly similar principles. In place of *yin* and *yang*, Galen spoke of medicinal plants as having a *dynameis*, or primary energetic quality, described as *hot* or *cold*, and *dry* or *moist*. For example, he classified the energetic nature of caraway seeds as *hot* and *dry*, and that of roses as *cool* and *moist*. And just as the Chinese physician would gear treatment of the patient toward re-establishing balance between *yin* and *yang*, so too would the Galenic herbalist attempt to restore harmony to the individual's *krasis* – their mixture of fluids, or "humours".

YIN AND YANG IN NATURE

While inseparable and complementary, *yin* and *yang* represent, at a fundamental level, the distinction between the material and substantial *(yin)*, and the immaterial and non-substantial *(yang)*. As polar tendencies rather than actual phenomena, *yin* and *yang* point toward the visible and solid *(yin)*, and invisible, dynamic *(yang)* aspects of the same entity. They cannot exist without each other, nor are capable of remaining fixed: they signify dynamic tension, interdependence, and change.

In terms of movement, any condensed, relatively stationary stage of nature is described as more *yin*, while any expansive, comparatively active, stage is more *yang*. One of the best examples of the inter-transformation of these stages is seen in

TO THE READER
A number of common anatomical terms appear in the text as italics, or begin, unusually, with an upper case letter. This is because words such as the Heart and *blood* refer, from an Oriental perspective, to more than simply an anatomical organ or fluid. They represent, in addition, specific energetic, psychological, and spiritual functions.

the water cycle. On land, water in its visible liquid state *(yin)* evaporates under the sun's heat *(yang)*, and rises upward as invisible vapour *(yang)*. When it cools, it condenses *(yin)* to form rain, descending *(yin)* to earth.

With regard to temperature and moisture, *yin* is more cool and moist, and *yang*, more warm and dry. Darkness, night, and Winter are all equated with *yin*; light, day, and Summer, with *yang*.

YIN AND YANG IN THE BODY

Just as, in the natural world, *yin* denotes the more substantial and *yang* the more rarefied, in the human body, *yin* pertains to anatomical structure – to the cells, tissues, and organs – while *yang*, in turn, relates to the body's energy, its vital force, and dynamic functioning.

Even within the structure of the body, however, we can see *yin* and *yang* polarities present. One of the most fundamental energetic divisions in Chinese medicine is between the body's more *yin*, nutritive "Interior", and its more *yang*, protective "Exterior".

The body's Interior houses the vital organs, and is sustained by the *Nutritive-Qi* . This is the type of *Qi-energy* that circulates along channels commonly known as "meridians". The body's Exterior includes the skin and muscles, and is controlled by the *Defensive-Qi*. This is the body's protective energy – the force that helps us to resist external pathogenic invaders such as bacteria and viruses.

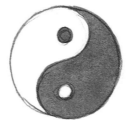

YIN

ENERGY CONDENSING
state substantial
velocity slower
direction descending
temperature cooler
moisture more moist
vital substances blood, body
fluids and essence
consciousness being

YANG

ENERGY EXPANDING
state non-substantial
velocity faster
direction rising
temperature warmer
moisture more dry
vital substances Qi and Mind
consciousness knowing

ENERGETIC FUNCTIONS OF YIN AND YANG

Understanding the energetic roles of *yin* and *yang* is the key to their therapeutic application – whether used in acupuncture, herbal medicine, or aromatherapy. Each function identified can be supported with particular essential oils, chosen with an eye to individual constitution and character. The primary function of the *yang* is to warm, energize, and stimulate, while that of the *yin* is to cool, moisten, relax, and promote sleep.

If an individual's *yang* energy is deficient, they are likely to feel chilly, tired, and unmotivated, and will benefit from warming, invigorating essential oils such as rosemary and ginger. These are oils that "tonify and *yang*" and "disperse *cold*". Rosemary and ginger essential oils are among those that promote the circulation of blood, stimulate digestive "fire", and counteract rheumatic pain of a *cold*, fixed, contracted nature.

However, the best results will be obtained by determining the precise organ(s) responsible for the deficient *yang-energy*, and selecting oils accordingly. If, for example, there is poor stamina and confidence, a weak and achy lower back, and frequent urination of a pale colour, it is likely that the *yang* of the Kidneys are weak. Such a condition is simply called *Kidney-yang* deficiency, and will benefit from thyme as well as ginger oil.

Yang energy can not only be weak and deficient but can also become excessive – especially where there has been a build-up of emotional stress. In place of fatigue, an *excess* of *yang* will produce restlessness, hyperactivity, and insomnia. As the function of the *yang* is to warm the body, an excess of *yang* can result in sensations of heat and thirst. In fact, another expression for "excess yang" is "heat".

Diagnostically, deficient *yang* (or *cold*) results in a pale tongue; excess *yang* (or *heat*) in a red tongue. Essential oils that reduce excess *yang* are inherently *cool* and relaxing, and include German chamomile and melissa. German chamomile oil is especially good for clearing *heat* from the

QI

Pronounced "chee", *Qi*, or *Qi-energy*, is the vital force of the body and mind. Like *yin* and *yang*, it can be seen at work not only in the body but in nature and the cosmos at large – the enlivening, formative principle behind all life processes. *Qi-energy* both moves and makes things move, and is the source of all bodily activity. Invisible, dynamic, and energizing, the *Qi* is an aspect of the *yang*.

Stomach and Liver, and therefore benefits problems that include gastritis, irritability, and headache. Melissa oil, in addition, clears *heat* from the Heart, and subsequently helps to ease cardiac palpitations.

Because the body's *yin* energy is cooling, moistening, and calming, a deficiency of *yin* will lead to heat, thirst, and restlessness. Although similar to the symptoms of excess *yang*, those of deficient *yin* have some important differences: feelings of heat are limited to the hands, feet, and chest; both heat and thirst are more predominant at night; and restlessness is underpinned by a sense of weakness.

Diagnostically, excess *yang* produces a swollen, red tongue, often with a yellow coating – while deficient *yin* results in a thin, red tongue, usually without a coating. Two of the best oils to strengthen the body's *yin* energy, and therefore to cool and relax, are rose and geranium.

Rose essential oil is indicated, in particular, for a deficiency of *Heart-yin*, and is therefore beneficial for a pattern of anxiety, thirst, insomnia, and night sweats. Geranium's ability to strengthen the *yin* of the Lungs makes it helpful for cases of a very dry cough.

However, like all essential oils, those of rose and geranium possess a range of energetic actions that are not just confined to their influence on the *yin*. These will be explored in Part II (see pp.49-129). Further functions of the *yang* include those of transforming, transporting, eliminating, and protecting, while those of the *yin* extend to absorbing, storing, generating, and sustaining.

PSYCHOLOGICAL ASPECTS OF YIN AND YANG

As *yang* is more abstract and exposed, it relates on a psychological level to conscious thought and analysis, and reflects the power of logic and inquiry. These capacities are strengthened by oils that increase concentration and alertness, such as rosemary and laurel.

In contrast, *yin* is darker, more hidden, and more earthly. It corresponds psychologically to feeling and impression, and to

ENERGIZING AND STIMULATING
While rosemary, ginger, and thyme essential oils are deeply energizing, peppermint and lemon may be described as stimulating, as their invigorating effect is quick and short-term. They mobilize the *Qi* rather than tonify (or strengthen) the *yang*, as they are cooling rather than warming.

the life both of the senses and emotions. These are generally enhanced by oils such as neroli and jasmine, both of which relax the mind but heighten our sensual awareness.

The ability to express oneself articulately and clearly is also more *yang*, while the capacity to be receptive and observant is more *yin*. Verbal self-expression is encouraged by oil of fennel, while emotional receptivity can be supported by rose.

In terms of personal drive, the more assertive and goal-orientated aspect of will-power may be considered more *yang*. Sharply focused and projected outward, it promotes a more structured, clearly planned approach to life. Will-power can be stimulated through the use of ginger and juniper berry oils, while rosemary promotes the ability to plan, helping to strengthen one's sense of purpose.

The more *yin* aspect of will-power gives us the ability to yield and adapt. Less clearly defined yet more inward and stable, it affords us the capacity for stillness and serenity. By reinforcing the *yin*, geranium oil can help to restrain and settle the will – to the benefit of those are driven and hyperactive.

The capacity for self-confidence is more *yang* in nature, in contrast to inner security, which is more *yin*. To enhance self-assurance, we might consider using thyme, while gaining a sense of emotional security is supported, in particular, by oil of rose.

THE RELATIVITY OF YIN AND YANG
It should always be remembered that yin and yang do not refer to two different constitutional or psychological types, but are simply ways of identifying the polarities that co-exist within each individual. The same is true of essential oils: no oil of itself can be labelled totally "yin" or "yang" – we can only say that an oil "strengthens yin" or "tonifies yang", just as it may have the capacity to "smooth the flow of Qi".

Yin & Yang

Yin	Yang	Yin	Yang
YIN AND YANG IN NATURE		**ENERGETIC FUNCTIONS OF YIN AND YANG**	
material	immaterial	calming	energizing
substantial	non-substantial	inhibiting	stimulating
matter	energy	cooling	warming
stasis	movement	absorbing	transforming
condensation	expansion	storing	transporting
centripetal movement	centrifugal movement	generating	eliminating
descending	ascending	moistening	protecting
darkness	light		
cold	warmth	**PSYCHOLOGICAL ASPECTS OF YIN AND YANG**	
moisture	dryness	feeling	thinking
space	time	impression	analysis
		sensation	idea
YIN AND YANG IN THE BODY		intuition	inspiration
structure	function	receptive	expressive
inferior	superior	observant	articulate
anterior	posterior	implicit	explicit
medial	lateral	yielding	assertive
Interior	Exterior	adaptable	single-minded
Nutritive-Qi	Defensive-Qi	spontaneous	structured
blood & body fluids	Qi	serenity	excitement
essence (Jing)	Mind (Shen)	inward security	outward confidence
		collective	individual
		being	knowing

The Five Elements

their seasons, organs, and spirits

Together with *yin* and *yang*, the theory of the Five Elements is one of the two main pillars of Oriental medicine (see diagram facing page). Comparatively more recent than *yin* and *yang*, it was first documented in China in the Warring States Period (476-221 BC). At first, the theories of *yin* and *yang* and the Five Elements co-existed independently, but the two systems began to merge, and in the Song Dynasty (AD 960-1279) the Five Elements first became employed in the diagnosis and treatment of illness.

The popularity of the Five Element system has waxed and waned throughout the history of Chinese medicine and culture. In some important books, such as *The Yellow Emperor's Classic of Internal Medicine* (*c.* 4th century BC), the Five Elements is a central feature, while in other texts it is not mentioned at all. However, there were periods during which the theory of the Five Elements was extremely popular, featuring in almost every part of Chinese culture. It was applied not only to medicine but to the natural sciences, the calendar, astrology, music, and politics. Everything was classified according to one of the Five Elements.

The Five Elements may be understood as five *phases* or *movements* of *yin* and *yang* energy. Rather than being elements in a literal sense, the images of water, wood, fire, earth, and metal represent natural forces that together form a dynamic whole.

The first of the Five Elements – Water – may be understood as energy in a condensed and relatively static *yin* phase, reflected by the dormancy of Wintertime and the night. Although Water represents a "floating" state of rest, it contains within itself the potential for growth and regeneration. It is therefore associated with the very source of life – with the procreative force and the will to survive.

The second Element – Wood – is indicative of energy in a rising and accelerating *yang* phase, as in the sense of awakening that comes with Springtime and morning. In this stage of transformation, the contained and latent forces of Water are aroused and given direction. The Wood Element is subse-

WOOD
rising yang
SEASON: *Spring*
TIME OF DAY: *morning*
BODILY ORGANS: *Liver & Gall Bladder*
SPIRIT: *Ethereal Soul (Hun)*
ROOT EMOTION: *Anger*
HIGHEST EXPRESSION: *Compassion*

FIRE
radiant yang
SEASON: *Summer*
TIME OF DAY: *midday*
BODILY ORGANS: *Heart, Pericardium, Small Intestines & Triple Heater*
SPIRIT: *Mind (Shen)*
ROOT EMOTION: *Joy*
HIGHEST EXPRESSION: *Love*

EARTH
descending yin
SEASON: *Late summer*
TIME OF DAY: *afternoon*
BODILY ORGANS: *Stomach & Spleen-pancreas*
SPIRIT: *Intellect (Yi)*
ROOT EMOTION: *Reflection*
HIGHEST EXPRESSION: *Empathy*

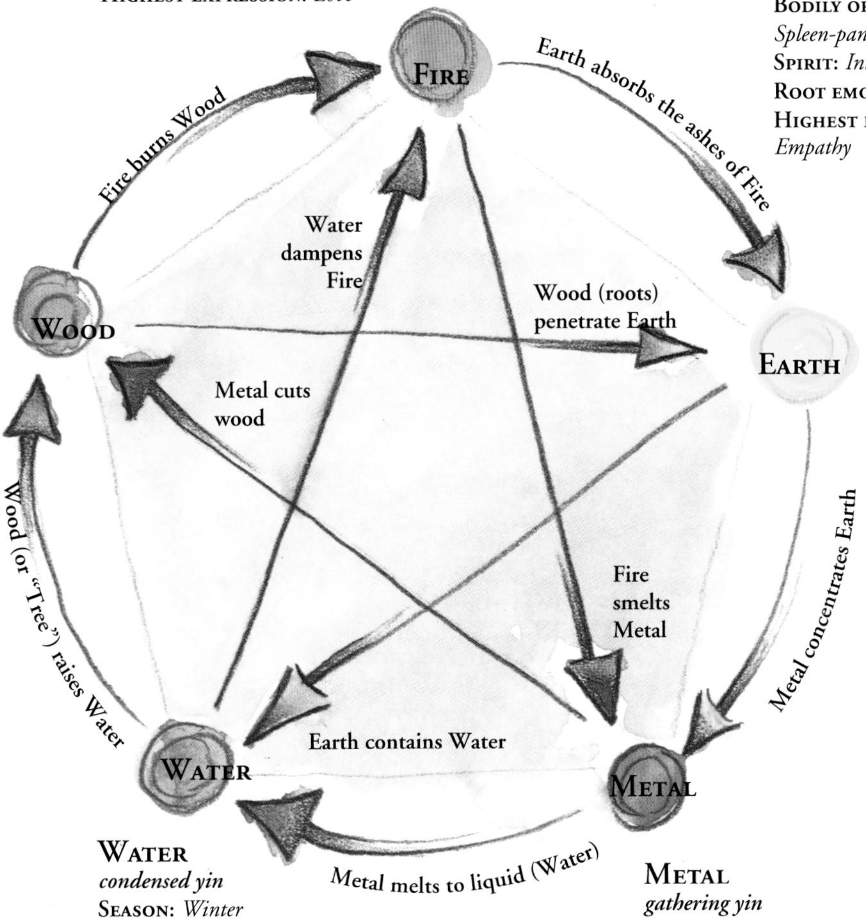

Fire burns Wood

Earth absorbs the ashes of Fire

Water dampens Fire

Wood (roots) penetrate Earth

Metal cuts wood

Fire smelts Metal

Wood (or "Tree") raises Water

Metal concentrates Earth

Earth contains Water

Metal melts to liquid (Water)

FIRE

WOOD

EARTH

WATER

METAL

WATER
condensed yin
SEASON: *Winter*
TIME OF DAY: *night*
BODILY ORGANS: *Kidneys & Bladder*
SPIRIT: *Will (Zhi)*
ROOT EMOTION: *Fear*
HIGHEST EXPRESSION: *Wisdom*

METAL
gathering yin
SEASON: *Autumn*
TIME OF DAY: *evening*
BODILY ORGANS: *Lungs & Large Intestines*
SPIRIT: *Bodily Soul (P'o)*
ROOT EMOTION: *Grief*
HIGHEST EXPRESSION: *Reverence*

quently associated with both movement and evolution.

The next Element is that of Fire – symbolic of energy at its most expansive and radiant, of *yang* at its zenith. It is the Element of Summer, of midday and noon. Fire takes the Wood Element's urge to move and evolve, and gives it *raison d'etre* – a "felt sense" of the ideal. Energy at its most refined and sensitive, it is associated with both conscious awareness and self-identity.

Fire is followed by the Element Earth – energy in its descending *yin* stage, in a general movement downward toward materialized form. Earth is predominant in late Summer and early Autumn, "the season of mellow fruitfulness", and in the afternoon. It takes the ideal inherent in Fire and makes it real, imbuing consciousness with concrete thought and Spirit with bodily form.

The fifth and final Element is that of Metal – energy in a gathering and synthesizing *yin* phase of transformation. Metal takes the formative nature of Earth and refines it, adding order and definition. The season of Metal is Autumn, and the time of day, evening – periods of quiescence and reflection. The Metal Element is also associated both with the urge to interact and the need to maintain distance.

The Five Elements are neither separate nor solid. They are phases of a continual energetic process that we can observe in potentially every aspect of life. The order in which I have presented them here illustrates their natural movement from *yin* to *yang* and back again. This is referred to as their Creation Cycle. While successive Elements nourish each other, those with an intermediate relationship impose restriction and constraint, and work to prevent imbalance. The Control Cycle, however, also has the potential for becoming a mutually destructive one. For example, if Water overflows, Fire will be extinguished; and if Wood grows too abundant, it will deplete the Earth of nutrients. Within the body/mind, pathological *Qi* often follows the Control Cycle, progressing from one organ to another along what ultimately becomes a cycle of destruction.

THE VALUE OF THE FIVE ELEMENTS

While *yin* and *yang* form the basis of the primary clinical aspect of Oriental medicine, the main value of the Five Element system lies in its psychological and spiritual dimension. Although *yin* and *yang* reveal a great deal about human psychology, it is the theory of the organs and their associated Elements that more accurately mirror the complexity of the human spirit.

So far, we have examined the Five Elements as fundamental forces of nature. As we proceed to consider in detail each Element, we shall see that we are provided with an immediate and easily applied "diagnostic" tool. The Five Elements afford a system of correspondences with immense potential for practical application, particularly in the field of psychological aromatherapy. And it is a system that relies on the use of all our faculties – on our logic, our feeling, our intuition, and the five senses.

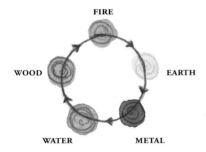

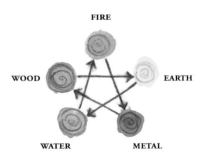

THE CREATION CYCLE
Applying the natural symbolism of the Elements, the Creation Cycle can be described as follows: Wood absorbs and raises Water within the tree or plant; Fire burns and consumes Wood; the ashes of Fire descend to the ground and are absorbed by Earth; from Earth are produced the concentration of ores that form Metal; Metal is smelted into the liquid state (Water).

THE CONTROL CYCLE
The mutually restraining nature of the Control Cycle may be expressed as follows: Water controls Fire through its power to dampen flames; Fire controls Metal through its capacity to smelt ore; Metal controls Wood through its ability to cut trees; Wood controls Earth through the fact that trees secure the soil; Earth controls Water through providing the foundation of streams and rivers.

Water

Winter - the Kidneys - the Will

The Water Element represents *Qi-energy* at its most consolidated and essential. Like the seed of a plant, it contains within itself both the potential for growth and the continuity of life. Water is a phase that appears outwardly to be dormant, yet is full of latent power – of energy gathered in states of germination, gestation, rest, and hibernation. Embodying the principle of fertility, Water signifies the life force in its primal condition, before it has been channelled and put to use. From an archetypal viewpoint, its main purpose is to *be* and endure, and, like the survival instinct, to *will.*

The main associated organ of the Water Element is the Kidneys. "The Kidneys call to life that which is dormant and sealed up; they are the natural organ for storing away, and they are the place where the secretions are lodged. The Kidneys influence the hair on the head and have an effect upon the bones. Within the *yin* the Kidneys act as the *lesser yin,* which permeates the climate of Winter." *(The Yellow Emperor's Classic of Internal Medicine)*

According to Chinese medicine, the Kidneys store the *essence* (or *Jing*), the genetic foundation of the individual. Formed at conception through the union of the parental *essences*, it is responsible for growth, reproduction, and development. The *essence* generates the marrow, which in turn produces the bone marrow, and fills the spinal cord and brain. The *essence* determines our constitutional strength and resistance to disease. Because it is inherited, it is fundamentally difficult to replenish, and is therefore considered precious – something to be carefully preserved. Problems that originate from a depleted *essence* include infertility, habitual miscarriage, bone deterioration, failing memory, and immune deficiency.

It is from the *essence* that the Kidneys produce the *Original-Qi.* The *Original-Qi* acts as catalyst for all bodily activity, and is one reason that the Kidneys are called the "root of *yin* and *yang*".

Apart from storing the *essence,* the other main role of the Kidneys is to *control water.* This we can more easily relate to

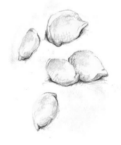

THE SEED OF THE ORANGE
The seed of a plant is a condensation of its fertility and procreative potential – qualities central to the Water Element.

its scientific anatomical function: that of separating excess body fluids and waste products from the blood. When *Kidney-Qi* is weak, and fails to control *water,* problems such as oedema (water retention) can occur. This condition may benefit from diuretic essential oils such as those of juniper and sweet fennel.

The Kidneys, in addition, house the aspect of the psyche known as the Will *(Zhi)* – the "spirit" from which we derive will-power, stamina, and a thirst for the enduring. Just as the *essence* oversees our growth and continuity, the Will is concerned with the unfolding of our destiny, and is the vehicle of self-fulfilment. Like the *essence,* the Will is "fertile" – the source of inventiveness and ingenuity.

When the Will is strong, and the Water Element is in harmony, we are determined, resourceful, and prudent, unwilling to dissipate energy on the superfluous or transitory. There is confidence and self-sufficiency, and a mind both penetrating and introspective.

When the Water Element is in disharmony, however, two main outcomes are possible. Either the Will is deficient, producing apathy and a feeling of powerlessness; or it is unrestrained, and the person is restless and driven.

In the first instance, where the Will is poorly rooted, there is a tendency to become easily discouraged, and to lack sufficient confidence to deal with difficult circumstances. Apprehensive and quickly overwhelmed, our urge in such a state is to avoid and retreat. Juniper is just one essential oil of benefit here. In the second instance, where the Will is hyperactive, the individual is unsettled and sometimes rash, unable to contain their personal drive. Described as a "workaholic", they demand too much of themselves – compelled by insecurity to succeed at any cost. Ultimately they may deplete themselves of both *Qi* and *yin,* succumbing to nervous "burn-out". Geranium oil is recommended here.

In both types of disharmony, the root emotion is fear – in the first instance, fear of the forces of the environment; in the second, fear of inadequacy and failure.

WISDOM
The highest expression of the Water Element is Wisdom. Wisdom is borne of a Mind that possesses a firm foundation – the result of a Will *(Zhi)* that is both deeply rooted and calmly judicious. Wisdom develops through knowledge that endures and is practised, and is expressed through action that is in harmony with the environment.

Wood

Spring - the Liver - the Ethereal Soul

The Wood Element encapsulates *Qi-energy* as it expands and rises, and like the shoot of a plant, embodies activated growth. In this phase, the life force latent in the Water Element is aroused and given direction; the Will *(Zhi)* of the Kidneys is channelled by a sense of purpose.

The Wood Element in nature is apparent not only in the coming to life of Spring but in the entire process of evolution. Overseeing the body's cycles and rhythms, it governs both our need to develop and ability to adapt. At a basic level, the Wood Element is therefore concerned with *movement* – with motivation, growth, and with the harmonious flow of life.

The principal organ of the Wood Element is the Liver. "The Liver has the functions of a military leader who excels in his strategic planning. . . [It] is the dwelling place of the soul, or spiritual part of man. The Liver influences the nails and is effective upon the sinews; it brings forth animal desires and vigour. The taste connected with the Liver is sour and the colour, green. Within *yang* the Liver acts as the *lesser yang,* which permeates the air in Spring." *(The Yellow Emperor's Classic of Internal Medicine)*

The Liver is responsible energetically for ensuring the smooth flow of *Qi-energy* throughout the body/mind. While the Lungs circulate *Qi* through the meridians, it is the job of the Liver to ensure that *Qi* moves freely and is spread evenly.

The Liver, in addition, has an important influence on the *blood.* It stores the *blood* in times of rest, releases it when we become active, and maintains, as with the *Qi,* its smooth and equable flow.

If the Liver falters in its action of "spreading" the *Qi,* the flow of *Qi-energy* will become impeded and irregular, and produce a condition known as *Qi-stagnation.* When the *Qi* stagnates, problems that involve spasm, distention, constriction, and pain are likely to arise. These include dyspepsia, constipation, headache, and painful menstruation. If the *blood* as well as the *Qi* has stagnated, the stasis is deeper, and so the pain is more severe.

COMPASSION

The highest expression of the Wood Element is Compassion. Compassion develops from a generosity of spirit, and the ability to "see" the human condition, unclouded by dogma or bitterness. Compassion is an expression of our ultimate power – the power that stems from the Universal Mind.

Stagnation of *Qi* and *blood* is also related to nervous tension and frustration. Tense, moody, and irritable conditions disrupt Liver function and constrict the flow of *Qi*. On the other hand, conditions of stagnant *Qi* can *produce* a state of nervous tension. Essential oils that smooth the flow of *Qi* tend to possess antispasmodic, analgesic and/or nerve relaxant properties – lavender being the most prominent example of these.

Just as the Kidneys house the Will *(Zhi)*, the Liver provides the residence of the Ethereal Soul *(Hun)* – the subtle, expansive aspect of the psyche that links the individual mind with the Universal Mind. The source of our dreams and visions, we derive from the Ethereal Soul a sense of purpose and direction in life. Not only is it associated with our inspirational dreams and visions but with sleeping, dreaming, and the faculty of sight.

The Ethereal Soul *(Hun)* provides the mind with "movement" and with adaptability, allowing it both the capacity for introspection and the power to project outward. Yet, like the Liver, it possesses a regulating function, helping to maintain emotional balance through curbing extremes of excitation and inertia.

As the foundation of the Ethereal Soul, the Liver is called the "resolute organ" – a storehouse of purpose, decisiveness and courage. It is the planner, organizer, and adventurer within us all.

In disharmony, the Wood Element can result in either a lack of purpose and ambition, or behaviour which is rigid, ruthless, and compulsive. The Liver's normal capacity for assertiveness – and for clearly expressed, well-controlled anger – can become suppressed in states of *Qi-stagnation*, and explosive when there is excess *yang* and *heat*.

Stagnant-Qi is also associated with the type of depression that comes of unexpressed anger and resentment. These feelings when suppressed and allowed to turn inward invariably afflict the Ethereal Soul, causing its natural state of hope and vision to become one of bitterness and despair.

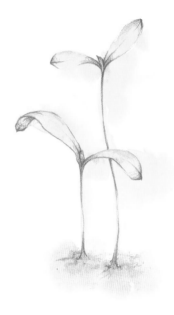

THE SPROUT OF THE ORANGE
The sprout, or young shoot, of a plant is an expression of the life force emerging from its latency, full of the upward movement that dominates the Wood Element.

Fire

Summer - the Heart - the Mind

The Fire Element is an expression of *Qi-energy* at its most exuberant, and like the flower, typifies radiance, attraction, and self-fulfillment. While the Water Element is the source of our basic drive, channelled and given direction by Wood, the Fire Element provides a "felt sense" of the ideal – a way of recognizing that which truly fulfils us. Without this, we may have energy and purpose, but will lack the self-understanding to succeed in finding joy.

The central organ of the Fire Element is the Heart. "The Heart is like the minister of the monarch who excels through insight and understanding. . . [It] is the root of life and causes versatility of spiritual faculties. Within *yang*, the principle of light and life, the Heart acts as the *Great Yang* which permeates the climate of Summer." *(The Yellow Emperor's Classic of Internal Medicine)*

Apart form its role of circulating and "governing" the *blood*, the Heart is the residence of the Mind *(Shen)* – of conscious awareness in all its forms. Directing the functions of thinking, feeling, memory, and imagination, the *Shen* is the focus of all mental-emotional activity, and is the source of self-awareness.

The word *Shen* is variously translated from the Chinese as "Mind" and "Spirit". However, if we take "Spirit" to indicate the sum-total of *all* aspects of the psyche, the *Shen* is more appropriately termed the "Mind", as it fulfils, in contrast, a specific role *within* the Spirit.

As the integrating factor of consciousness and perception, the *Shen* unites the disparate aspects of the Self, and through the Heart – the "minister of the monarch" – orchestrates the various "spirits" of the organs. It serves this function through an inherent sense of harmony and perfection, and a subsequent power to maintain balance.

As the source of emotional harmony, it is also through the Heart that we experience warmth and tenderness. Just as the heart has always been a symbol of love, so according to Oriental medicine it is the organ of love and affection – both as receiver and giver of emotional warmth.

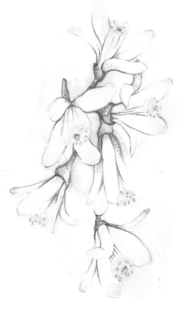

THE FLOWER OF THE ORANGE
The flower of a plant is often its supreme expression, and represents the full unfolding of its individual uniqueness – a process that is symbolized by the Fire Element.

The focus of sensitivity and feeling, the equanimity of the Heart and Mind is fundamentally responsible for ensuring a well-integrated and contented emotional life – as well as a balanced mind. Most psychological problems will subsequently involve, at least to some degree, an imbalance within the Fire Element.

The enthusiasm and spontaneity that reflects the Heart in harmony can become, when under stress, a feeling of nervousness and agitation. Moreover, the natural sensitivity and passion of the Fire Element, if it blazes out of control, can result in an individual who easily becomes over-excited and is quickly hurt. Nervous exhaustion and insomnia are often the consequences.

These types of imbalance are more typical of individuals who are energetically *hot* by nature, often due to excess *yang* energy. They will invariably benefit from essential oils that cool and calm the Heart and nerves, and reduce excessive *yang*. Some of the most important of these are lavender, melissa, and neroli oils. When the Heart is deficient in *yang*, however, a different picture emerges. Rather than over-excitement and agitation, there is a lack of enthusiasm and *joie de vivre*. The naturally warm and vibrant state of the Mind *(Shen)* is lost to apathy and despondency. These are occasions for using oils such as jasmine.

Disharmonies of a Fire nature can also be characterized by problems of self-identity. These may manifest either as self-centredness and selfishness, or, more problematically, as poor self-image and low self-esteem. In this sense, the Heart represents not only our relationships with others but the understanding and compassion that we have for *ourselves*. Rose oil may be used to enhance love and acceptance for both oneself and others.

Anxiety is a state common to all types of constitution – whether *hot* or *cold, excess* or *deficient*. Described in terms of Oriental medicine as a disturbance of the Mind *(Shen)*, the appropriate oils vary, and are discussed in Part III (see pp.142-5).

LOVE
The highest expression of the Fire Element is Love. Real love radiates from the centre of our being, and has the quality of an embrace or smile. Love is said by poets to be inherently pure and perfect – and can never be shamed, only wounded. Love possesses the power to restore faith and harmony, and has been the ultimate teaching of many spiritual masters.

Earth

late Summer - the Spleen-Pancreas - the Intellect

The Earth Element represents *Qi-energy* in a formative and concretizing mode, and is concerned with generating and maintaining physical form. Like the fruit of the plant, it embodies nourishment and abundance, the ripening of the life force into the palpable and sustaining. It is supported in these processes by the power to absorb and transform, and is associated on a mental level with learning, thinking, and analysis. According the Creation Cycle of the Five Elements, the Earth Element follows Fire – reflecting its role in furnishing the Mind *(Shen)* with the capacity for concrete thought.

The organs associated with the Earth Element are the Spleen-pancreas and Stomach. "These organs influence the lips and the shape of the flesh and muscles. The flavour connected with these organs is sweet and the colour is yellow. They belong to the *yin* which permeates the climate of the earth." *(The Yellow Emperor's Classic of Internal Medicine)*

The principal energetic function of the Spleen-pancreas and Stomach is to transform and transport. As the central organs of digestion, they are responsible for the transformation of food and drink into *Qi, body fluids,* and *blood.* Along with the Kidneys and Lungs, the Spleen and Stomach are the key providers of strength and vitality. When, due to deficiency of *Qi-energy* and *yang,* their transformation function becomes impaired, symptoms of sluggish digestion ensue. These include a lack of appetite, epigastric distention, dyspepsia, hiccough, and flatulence. Essential oils such as cardamom, fennel, and thyme may be used to strengthen the Spleen-pancreas and stimulate the Stomach.

When the Spleen and Stomach fail to fully transform food and fluids, excessive moisture can accumulate in the body, producing conditions of *dampness* and *phlegm* (mucus). *Dampness* is characterized by a feeling of distention in the epigastrium and lower abdomen, by heaviness of the head and limbs, and by general lassitude. It is frequently associated with conditions of obesity and lymphatic congestion, and benefits from oils such as grapefruit and juniper.

The influence of the Spleen-pancreas on the *blood* is two-

EMPATHY
The highest expression of the Earth Element is Empathy. This emotion results from a perspective of oneness, and, like the love of a parent for its child, reflects the ability to make no final distinction between self and other. It is from empathy that we derive both conscience and a sense of community – as well as the power to truly "hear" and heal another.

fold. As the organ responsible for the transformation of food essences into *blood*, the Spleen is considered the origin of *blood*, ensuring its ability to nourish and sustain. In addition, the Spleen is said to *control* the *blood* – that is, to hold it securely in the vessels. If the *Qi* of the Spleen is deficient, the blood vessels can lose their tone and become weak, resulting in problems such as haemorrhoids.

Of the five "spirits", the Spleen houses the Intellect *(Yi)*, the aspect of the psyche responsible for thinking, concentrating, studying, and memorizing. Just as the organs of the Earth Element oversee the digestion of food, so too are they concerned with the absorption and analysis of ideas and information. If the *yang* and *Qi-energy* of the Spleen is deficient, concentration can become impaired and thinking dulled. Just as weakness of the Spleen produces fullness and congestion on a bodily level, it results in overthinking and mental churning on an intellectual one. In this instance, essential oils such as frankincense and lemon may be employed to settle and clarify the Intellect *(Yi)*, and to alleviate worry and mental confusion.

Essentially nurturing, the Earth Element on an emotional level is associated with caring, support, and sympathy, and with issues of commitment and community. The person with an abundance of Earth energy is empathetic and loyal, keen to provide security. An imbalance of Earth, however, can manifest in an overprotective attitude – as in the person who continually worries about their children, neglecting their own needs. For this, lemon oil can be of benefit.

A different type of Earth imbalance is characterized by dependency and neediness. Here, the overdeveloped urge to sympathize becomes an excessive *need* for sympathy and support – as a lack of sufficient Earth depletes one's ability to contain and help oneself. The principal oils for this type of problem are marjoram and vetiver.

THE FRUIT OF THE ORANGE
The fruit of a plant is generally sweet, fleshy, and nourishing, and ensures that its seeds are adequately transported for the purposes of germination. All these characteristics belong to the Earth Element.

Metal

Autumn - the Lungs - the Bodily Soul

The Metal Element represents both the interchange and synthesis of *Qi-energy*. The functions of the leaf of the plant provide a good example of this activity, incorporating, as they do, the processes of transpiration and photosynthesis – the exchange of vital gases, and the transmutation of solar into nutritive energy. As the Element of dynamic exchange and interaction – and of the extraction of energy from the environment – Metal is also linked to the concept of boundary. It is the physical and metaphorical "skin" through which we "take in" and "let go".

The principal organ of the Metal Element is the Lungs. "The Lungs are the origin of breath and the dwelling of the animal spirits or inferior soul. The Lungs influence the body hair and have their effect upon the skin. The Lungs act as the *Great Yin* which permeates the climate in Autumn." *(The Yellow Emperor's Classic of Internal Medicine)*

As the central organ of respiration, the Lungs are said to "govern" the *Qi*, inhaling the "pure *Qi*" of air and exhaling the "dirty *Qi*" of metabolism. They are responsible, in addition, for the synthesis of the *Nutritive-* and *Defensive-Qi*, formed from the fusion of *Air-* and *Food-Qi*. The role of the *Nutritive-Qi* is to sustain and nourish, and is distributed by the Lungs to all bodily organs (via the meridians); the *Defensive-Qi* is dispersed round the periphery of the body to protect it from pathogenic invasion.

The Lungs are crucial, therefore, for ensuring the vitality of both body and mind. If Lung function is impaired, there will be tiredness, shortness of breath, and a feeling of melancholy. If, in addition, there is an insufficient supply of *Defensive-Qi*, frequent colds are likely to occur. Eucalyptus and tea tree oils can be used to strengthen the Lungs and respiration, and enhance the power of the immune system.

If there is both a deficiency of *Lung-Qi* and a weakness of the Spleen-pancreas, the production of *phlegm*, or mucus, is common. Whether nasal or bronchial, *phlegm* can take a clear, white, and copious form – indicative of *cold phlegm* –

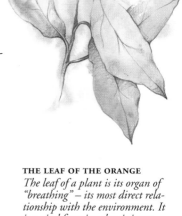

THE LEAF OF THE ORANGE
The leaf of a plant is its organ of "breathing" – its most direct relationship with the environment. It is a vital function that is inseparable from the Metal Element.

or a sticky, yellow form – characteristic of *hot phlegm*.

While the Liver is said to house the Ethereal Soul *(Hun)*, the Lungs provide the residence of the Bodily Soul *(P'o)*. The *P'o* is the bodily or "animal" aspect of the human soul, and forms the physical, more *yin* counterpart of the *Hun*. The Bodily Soul is primarily instinctive and sensory in nature, and provides us with the capacity for physical sensation and touch, as well as taste, smell, sight, and hearing. It also affords an animal-like sixth sense, which helps to fulfil, on a subtle level, the Metal Element's function of protection.

The process of breathing can be viewed as the pulsating of the Bodily Soul *(P'o)*, which relies for its inherent vibrancy on the vitality of the *Qi*. On the other hand, the *Qi* and the breath are dependent on the health of the Bodily Soul.

Living as it does in the moment, the Bodily Soul is affect-ed, in particular, by feelings of regret, remorse, and a lingering sense of loss. These emotions, in turn, can obstruct the orderly rhythmic function of the Lungs as they "take in" and "let go", reflecting an inability psychologically to fully accept and relinquish. A Bodily Soul that is constricted by a persistent feeling of grief can therefore result in chronic fatigue and breathing difficulties.

As the "skin" of the body/mind – its sensitive, interactive boundary – the Metal Element is also concerned with issues of relationship and individuality. Those with a *strong* Metal Element may be by nature reserved, yet will instinctively seek out interaction and communication as a source of stimula-tion and insight. If the Metal Element is afflicted, however, the individual is likely instead to feel psychologically exposed and vulnerable, and will tend to withdraw and isolate them-selves.

Overall, the Metal Element in harmony promotes order, communication, and positivity, while under stress can result in constriction, withdrawal, and pessimism.

REVERENCE

The highest expression of the Metal Element is Reverence. This emotion conveys the recog-nition of that which inspires and transforms – an honouring of the distinctive and sacred. Through Reverence we regain a true perspective of our place in the Universe, yet are renewed by its power to deepen and purify.

	WATER	**WOOD**
YIN/YANG PHASE	condensed *yin*	rising *yang*
SEASON	Winter	Spring
TIME OF DAY	night	morning
COLOUR	blue/black	green
LIFE FUNCTIONS	procreation survival	evolution & adaptation movement & growth
BODILY ORGANS	Kidneys & Bladder	Liver & Gall Bladder
SPIRIT	Will *(Zhi)*	Ethereal Soul *(Hun)*
BODILY TISSUE	bones	tendons & ligaments
SENSE ORGAN	ears	eyes
BODILY MANIFESTION	head hair	nails
SOUND OF VOICE	groaning	shouting
FUNCTIONS OF MAIN ORGAN	- Stores the genetic essence *(Jing)* - Controls water	- Ensures the smooth flow of *Qi* and *blood* - Stores the *blood*
ROOT EMOTION	Fear	Anger
PSYCHOLOGICAL FUNCTIONS	will-power, stamina, ingenuity	purpose, foresight, adaptability
IN HARMONY	determined, resourceful, wise	motivated, well-organized, easy-going
IN DISHARMONY	apathetic, unconfident, apprehensive, restless, driven, insecure	tense, frustrated, angry, rigid, repressive, compulsive
HIGHEST EXPRESSION	Wisdom	Compassion
ESSENTIAL OILS	cedarwood, geranium, ginger, juniper berry, thyme (caraway, cypress, jasmine sandalwood, vetiver)	bergamot, chamomile, everlasting, grapefruit, sweet orange, yarrow (lavender, melissa, neroli, peppermint, spikenard)

FIRE	EARTH	METAL
radiant *yang*	descending *yin*	gathering *yin*
Summer	late Summer	Autumn
midday	afternoon	evening
red	yellow	white
self-realization idealization & fulfilment	concretization nourishment	transmutation & synthesis interchange
Heart & Pericardium	Spleen-pancreas & Stomach	Lungs & Large Intestines
Mind *(Shen)*	Intellect *(Yi)*	Bodily Soul *(P'o)*
blood vessels	muscles	skin
tongue	mouth	nose
complexion	lips	body hair
laughing	singing	weeping
- Houses the Mind *(Shen)* -Governs (circulates) the *blood*	- Transforms & transports *Qi* - Controls the *blood*	- Governs *Qi* & respiration - Distributes *Qi* & body fluids
Joy	Reflection	Grief
awareness, self-identity, harmony and love	concentration, cognition, sympathy	boundary, instinct, interaction
sensitive, well-integrated, joyful	attentive, thoughtful, supportive	communicative, vital, positive
nervous, anxious, agitated, hypersensitive, despondent, lacking self-esteem	vague, confused, worried, over-protective, dependent self-doubting	melancholic, regretful, pessimistic, vulnerable, unresponsive, remote
Love	Empathy	Reverence
jasmine, laurel, lavender, melissa, neroli, palmarosa, rose, rosemary, spikenard, ylang ylang (coriander seed, ginger, lemon, patchouli, tea tree)	benzoin, cardamom, coriander seed, fennel, frankincense, lemon, sweet marjoram, myrrh, patchouli, peppermint, sandalwood, vetiver (geranium, grapefruit)	cypress, clary sage, eucalyptus, hyssop, pine, tea tree, thyme (frankincense, juniper berry, sweet marjoram, myrrh, yarrow)

Essential oils and Astrology
the symbolic relationship of plants and planets

In addition to classifying plants energetically – according to their *temperature* and *moisture* – it became customary among certain Western schools to assign them to astrological signs and planets. The link between astrology and medicine is ancient, forming part of the medical philosophy of Hippocrates (460-377 BC), known as the "father of medicine". Hippocrates investigated medical records discovered in Chaldea, where both physical disease and its cure were closely linked to planetary cycles. Hippocrates came to believe that a good physician had to have a basic knowledge of astrology, due to its importance as a diagnostic tool.

The Swiss physician and astrologer Paracelsus (AD 1490-1541) integrated Hippocratic medicine with the practice of alchemy. Paracelsus not only attributed each body part to a zodiacal sign, and each organ to a planet, but catalogued the planetary "rulership" of many herbal medicines, precious stones, and colours. He looked to the individual horoscope to reveal both the cause and cure of disease, believing its origin to be of an emotional-spiritual nature.

Nicholas Culpeper (1616-54) is perhaps the best-known traditional herbalist-astrologer. Like Paracelsus, he ascribed each medicinal plant to a specific astrological planet, attempting to maintain the credence of medical astrology with the increasingly skeptical College of Physicians.

The astrological Sun is traditionally associated with mythological deities that include the Babylonian Shamash, the Egyptian Ra, and the Greek Apollo. The source of light and life, the Sun is naturally *hot* and *dry* in nature, and symbolizes the *yang* energy of the body/mind. It is linked to the heart and circulatory system, the thymus gland, and overall resistance to disease. Aromatic plants that are "ruled" by the Sun include rosemary, laurel, and frankincense. The focus of their subtle action is upon the Self – in both its "egoic" and "higher" aspects.

The Moon is linked to the goddesses of fertility and wisdom – to the Greek Artemis and Roman Diana. *Cool, moist,* and essentially feminine, the Moon reflects the *yin* energy of the body/mind. It "governs" digestion and nourishment, the pancreas and the mammary glands. Affiliated plants include jasmine, coriander, and clary sage – aromatics that enhance both creativity and intuition.

The planet Mercury is represented by the messenger gods – ancient lords of knowledge. These include the Egyptian Thoth, the Greek Hermes, and the Roman Mercurius. Mercury is related to the nervous system, the thyroid gland, and to speech and hearing. It is associated with fennel and caraway, as their focus is on movement and stability.

Venus is the planet of love and beauty, embodied, for example, by the Greek goddess Aphrodite. Venus pertains to the skin, the parathyroid gland, and the female reproductive system. It rules all traditional Herbs of Love – including rose, geranium, lemon, and benzoin. While Venus is *cool* and *moist*, Mars is *hot* and *dry*, and is symbolized mythologically by the warrior gods – the Egyptian Horus and the Greek Aries. Mars is reflected in the blood, the muscles, the adrenal glands, and the male reproductive system. It is associated with invigorating, pungent and "purging" oils – ginger and juniper among them.

Jupiter is personified by kingly gods – by the Greek Zeus, for example. *Warm* and *moist*, it represents bodily growth, the liver, and the anterior pituitary gland. It tends to rule aromatics that promote a sense of expansion and positivity – such as hyssop and orange oils.

The last of the traditional planets is the *cold, dry* Saturn – represented by Kronos, Greek lord of time. It governs the bones, the posterior pituitary gland, and the ageing process. Symbolic of stability and endurance, it is an appropriate emblem for cedarwood oil.

THE ASTROLOGICAL PLANETS
Each astrological planet symbolizes a psychological archetype, and according to medical astrology, represents a particular bodily system. Pictured below, in a clockwise direction, are the glyphs of the seven traditional planets: the Sun, the Moon, Mercury, Venus, Mars, Jupiter, and Saturn.

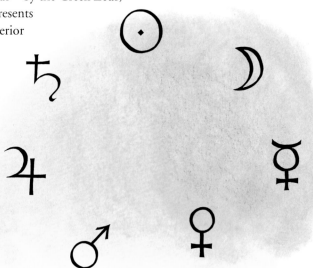

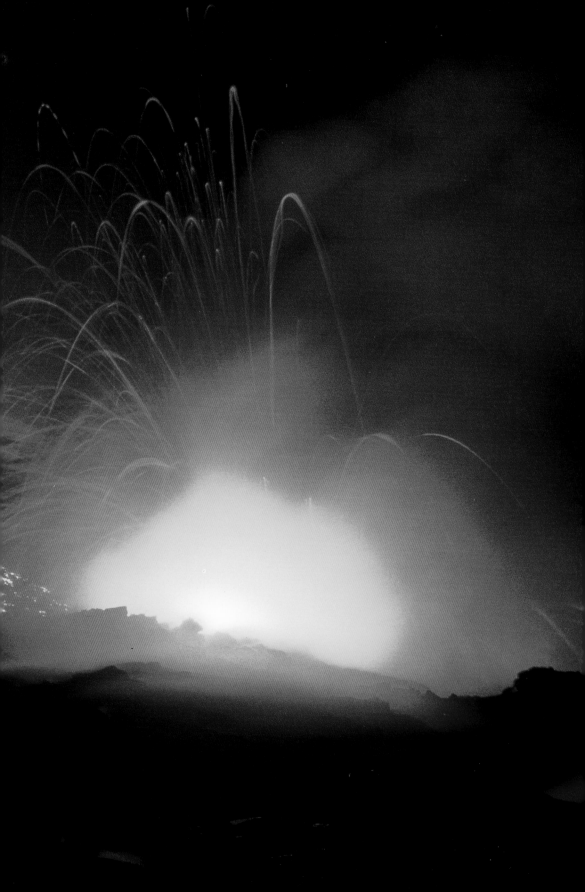

Part Two
Materia Aromatica

THE RADIANCE OF THE VOLCANO'S EMERGING LAVA
"Fire generates Earth"

In order to tap the full potential of aroma-therapy, we should try to understand each essential oil as we would a friend. The unique therapeutic "signature" of each essential oil is the reflection of its vital force – the dominating life-principle that Paracelsus, the alchemist-physician, called the *archeus*, known in Oriental medicine as the *Qi*.

Subtle and immaterial in nature, it is only possible to apprehend the *Qi* of an essential oil through an appreciation of the details of its individual make-up – its botanical structure and habitat, chemistry and aroma, history and tradition, and its properties and uses. Only a close and careful observation of the oil's *persona*, or "mask", will allow us to perceive its inner "character". For example, consideration of an essential oil's aroma affords us – from the perspective of Oriental medicine – some important insights into therapeutic nature. The sweet aroma produces a relaxing, nourishing, and harmonizing effect. Restoring the Spleen-pancreas and calming the Heart, it is predominant in both resinous oils such as benzoin, and floral ones like ylang ylang. The pungent scent, in contrast, is penetrating and dispersing. It is prevalent in essential oils that activate the *Lung-Qi* and clear *phlegm*, including those of eucalyptus and pine. The spicy aroma is similar in nature, though more *warm* and invigorating. Clearly present in ginger – yet discernible in coriander and other essential oils – it promotes blood circulation and helps to uplift the Mind *(Shen)*.

Oils with a sour or citrus quality are, like lemon and grapefruit, cooling, cleansing, and astringent. The bitter taste and aroma, on the other hand, is essentially a stimulant of the *Qi*, helping it to move, transform, and eliminate. It benefits the Liver, Kidneys, and Heart, and is strong in both juniper and German chamomile oils. The energetic influence of further aromas – earthy, woody, or floral – are interpreted where they appear in the *Materia Aromatica* that follows.

Benzoin

soothing Ø stabilizing Ø nurturing

The name "benzoin" is derived from the Arabic *luban-jawi*, meaning "incense from Java". Benzoin oil is derived from a large tropical tree that grows to a height of 20 metres (65 feet). It has pale-green, hairy, ovate leaves, flat, hard-shelled fruits, and drooping clusters of fleshy flowers, yellow or white in colour. Growing throughout Southeast Asia, particularly in Thailand and Indonesia, the trees are ready to be tapped for resin seven years after planting.

Tapping the tree involves making incisions into its trunk, from which a sap exudes and solidifies on exposure to air. The resulting reddish-brown gum is treated with solvents such as alcohol to produce a lighter *resinoid* – which is not, strictly speaking, an essential oil. It is possible – even preferable – to buy benzoin in its unadulterated solid state, and melt it as required by placing the bottle in hot water first.

Benzoin has been used for centuries in the Far East both as an incense and medicine, and was employed by Chinese physicians for respiratory and urinary complaints of a *cold, damp* nature. A powdered form of the gum resin was popular in Ancient Greece and Rome as an aromatic fixative for pot-pourris. "Gum benjamin", as it was called in medieval Europe, became best known as the key ingredient of "Friar's Balsam". It was applied to sore, cracked skin and vaporized and inhaled for respiratory complaints. Indeed, in France it became known as *baume pulmonaire*, or pulmonary balsam, as the resin was burned and inhaled to soothe chronic coughs and bronchitis.

Benzoin's sweet, *warm*, and resinous base-note characteristics associate it strongly with the Earth Element. Indeed, it is one of the most important essential oils for deficient *yang* energy of the Spleen-pancreas; benefiting lethargy, *cold* limbs, poor appetite, and abdominal distention. It may be combined, for this pattern, with oils of cardamom, ginger, and cedarwood. Benzoin oil's anti-infectious properties also make it useful for urinary infections of a *cold, damp* nature. This includes cystitis and urethritis characterized by cramping pain and pale, cloudy urine.

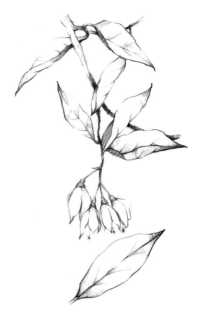

BENZOIN
Styrax benzoin
FAMILY: *Styraceae*
PARTS USED: *The gum*
AROMA: *Resinous, balsamic, sweet, rich & vanilla-like*
ENERGY: *Warm & dry*
MAIN ELEMENT: *Earth*
PROPERTIES: *Anticatarrhal, anti-infectious, astringent, calmative, carminative, cicatrisant, diuretic (mild), expectorant, vulnerary*
SAFETY DATA: *Non-toxic; non-irritant*

A soothing expectorant, benzoin oil can be used to benefit chronic bronchitis and asthma of a *cold,* catarrhal nature, with mucus that is clear or white in colour. Its balsamic quality makes it particularly useful for relieving painful coughs and sore throats, especially where there is hoarseness and loss of voice. For laryngitis, it may be combined with oils of eucalyptus, tea tree, and clary sage, and applied in a base cream to the throat.

The combination of benzoin's balsamic and vulnerary (wound-healing) properties make it indicated for chapped skin, chilblains, frostbite, and cuts. Made into an ointment, benzoin is excellent for protecting the hands against cold, wet weather conditions.

Psychologically, benzoin oil is generally considered to be a "sedative" essential oil. More specifically, it is indicated for the overthinking and worry that result from deficient *yang* energy of the Spleen, the Earth Element organ that houses the Intellect *(Yi)*. Rich, sweet, and comforting, benzoin softens the mind's "sharp edges", and gently "grounds" awareness abstracted by troubled thoughts. It is particularly good for nervous anxiety and worry made worse by exhaustion.

Benzoin oil can also be of benefit whenever a stabilizing, consolidating influence is required, as in times of physical and emotional upheaval. It has for this reason been recommended for those who pursue "spiritual journeys", as it helps to steady and focus the mind for meditation, contemplation, and prayer. It has thus remained an important ingredient of incense for Buddhist and Hindu temples.

The ability of benzoin to help calm, centre, and reassure also makes it suitable for those who feel emotionally needy and neglected – feelings that can denote a deficiency of Earth. Associated with the astrological Venus, planet of love, its warm, sweet, nourishing quality feeds and inspires our ability to nurture, to comfort both self and others.

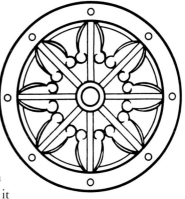

THE WHEEL OF TRUTH
Also known as the "Indestructible Wheel of the Cosmos", the Buddhist Wheel of Truth (Dharmachakra) conveys benzoin oil's ability to both stabilize the Intellect (Yi) in the face of life's vicissitudes, and centre the Spirit on the hub of Truth.

Bergamot

release ⊘ relax ⊘ uplift

Bergamot oil – like those of orange, lemon, and grapefruit – is obtained from the cold expression of the rind of a citrus fruit. The rather small bergamot fruits are picked for distillation while still unripe and green, the product of a variety of bitter orange tree. The tree, which grows to a height of five metres (16 feet), has dark-green ovate leaves and fragrant star-shaped flowers. Originating in tropical parts of Asia, the tree is grown in southern Italy, Sicily, and the Ivory Coast.

The bergamot tree is said to have been imported from the Canary Islands to Spain by Christopher Columbus. From there it was introduced into Calabria, in southern Italy. It is still uncertain where the name "bergamot" originates. It may be named after the Italian city Bergamo in Lombardy, where the oil was first produced, or may even have derived from the shape of the fruit, which resembles the bergamot pear.

Bergamot oil was an important remedy in Italian folk medicine, and from the 16th century onward appeared in a number of European herbals as an antiseptic and febrifuge. In Napoleonic times it was especially popular as a perfume, and became a key ingredient of the classic toilet water eau-de-Cologne.

It is now possible to buy bergamot oil that is free of furocoumarins, the group of constituents that heighten the skin's sensitivity to sunlight. These compounds are classified as "phototoxic", as they can penetrate the nuclei of skin cells and cause harmful reactions when the skin is exposed to ultra-violet light.

Like all the citrus oils, bergamot is essentially cooling, refreshing, and antidepressive. Its gently relaxing, yet distinctly uplifting, effect is the result not only of its beautifully fresh, fruity-floral aroma but the fact that it smooths the flow of *Qi-energy*. This energetic property of the oil relates directly to its ability to harmonize *Liver-Qi*, the function of which is to maintain the free and even flow of vital energy throughout the body/mind.

When the smooth flow of *Qi-energy* becomes disrupted and affects processes of digestion – a common result of both

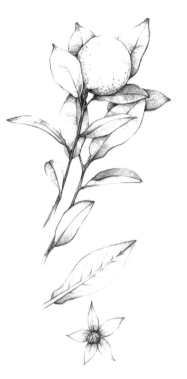

BERGAMOT
Citrus aurantium ssp. bergamia
FAMILY: *Rutaceae*
PARTS USED: *The rind*
AROMA: *Sweet & fruity; fresh & citrus; green & slightly floral*
ENERGY: *Cool & dry*
MAIN ELEMENT: *Wood*
PROPERTIES: *Antibacterial, antidepressive, anti-infectious, antispasmodic, calmative, carminative, digestive stimulant, stomachic*
SAFETY DATA: *Phototoxic: avoid exposure to direct sunlight or sunbed rays for 12 hours following application of the diluted essential oil to the skin*

over-eating and nervous tension – abdominal distention, indigestion, and colic can occur. Combined with oils such as coriander, chamomile, and fennel, bergamot will help to rectify these problems through releasing and circulating stagnant *Qi* in the stomach and intestines. Bergamot oil is particularly indicated for *nervous* indigestion and loss of appetite due to emotional stress.

While bergamot oil may also be used for genito-urinary infections and skin disorders, its principal therapeutic value rests with its regulating effect on the nervous system. Here, its deeply calming yet gently toning action contributes both to its antispasmodic nature and to its ability to relieve nervous depression and anxiety. These effects have been well documented by the Italian researcher Paolo Rovesti, who noted important psychological benefits for patients under psychiatric care.

Bergamot oil's psychological action depends, once again, on its ability to disperse stagnant *Qi-energy*. This condition can manifest as tension, irritability, and frustration, and if never released or "processed" can eventually result in depression. Depression due to stagnant *Qi-energy* is therefore the result of accumulated stress or repressed emotion. The emotion most often involved is that of unexpressed anger – the key emotion of the Liver and Wood Element. Anger and frustration turned inward oppress the Ethereal Soul *(Hun)* and block the free-flow of *Qi*, depressing mind and Spirit.

Like lavender, bergamot oil encourages the release of pent-up feelings – feelings that can lead not only to depression but to insomnia, anxiety, and sudden mood swings. It helps, in addition, to redirect nervous energy away from unproductive or addictive behaviour, helping us to rediscover spontaneity and optimism. Bergamot oil helps us to relax and "let go".

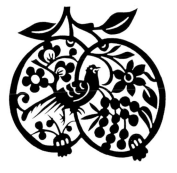

THE MAGPIE
The Chinese term for the magpie, pictured in these fruits, literally means "bird of joy". It is a bird whose chattering voice is considered to be light-hearted and to bear good fortune. It evokes the happy, carefree, and uninhibited feelings that are inspired by bergamot oil.

Caraway

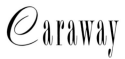

steadfast determination ∅ confident commitment

Caraway is a biennial herb, growing to a height of 30-60 centimetres (11 to 22 inches), with feathery, pinnate leaves and umbels of minute white flowers. The flowers bear fruits that ripen in autumn into the ribbed oblong seeds that contain the essential oil. As a member of the carrot or *Umbelliferae* family, caraway is one of a tribe of aromatic seed-producing herbs that include fennel, coriander, and cumin.

Caraway is native to Europe, Siberia, and North Africa, and is grown commercially in the Netherlands and eastern Europe. Cultivated mainly for its culinary uses, the seed is a characteristic flavouring in central European cooking, where it is used to season breads, cakes, cheeses, and vegetable dishes. The common name "caraway" derives from the Arabic word for "seeds", *al-karwiya*.

Judging from the discovery of fossilized caraway seeds amongst the debris of the Neolithic Swiss lake-dwellers, it is likely that the plant has been used by humankind for some 8,000 years. Caraway was utilized in Ancient Egypt as a ritual aromatic and food ingredient, while the Romans dipped the seeds in sugar to make "comfits" – served after meals to aid digestion and relieve flatulence.

The Greek physician Galen, in his text *On Simple Remedies* (AD165), classified the seed as *hot* and *dry* "in the third degree", reflecting the oil's spicy, warming, stimulating nature. Nicholas Culpeper associated the plant with the astrological Mercury. The planet of movement and thinking, it reflects the ability of these oils to circulate vital energy, stimulate digestion, and invigorate the mind. Culpeper says that caraway seeds are "conducing to all cold griefs of the head, stomach and bowels".

In terms of Oriental medicine, caraway oil promotes the flow of *Qi-energy* in the Stomach and intestines, alleviating spasm and encouraging peristalsis (smooth muscle functioning). It is indicated for abdominal distention, indigestion, nausea, belching, and flatulence. Caraway oil, for these conditions, may be blended with those of fennel, orange, and marjoram.

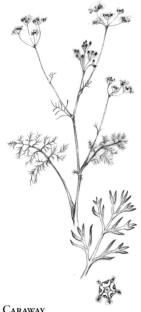

Caraway
Carum carvi
Family: *Umbelliferae (Apiaceae)*
Parts used: *The seeds*
Aroma: *Strong, spicy, bittersweet & warm; reminiscent of aniseed*
Energy: *Hot & dry*
Main element: *Earth (& Water)*
Properties: *Antibacterial, anti-catarrhal, anti-infectious, antispasmodic, aperitive, carminative, digestive stimulant, diuretic (mild), emmenagogic, expectorant, stomachic, general tonic, vermifuge*
Safety data: *Non-toxic; mild irritant of the mucous membranes*

Hot, sweet, and invigorating, caraway oil, in addition, strengthens the *yang* energy of the Spleen-pancreas. It promotes the Spleen's energetic function of transformation, helping to prevent the formation of *dampness* (excessive moisture), as well as the accumulation of *phlegm*. Like juniper and fennel oils, it is suitable for individuals who tend to be overweight, tired, and chilly by nature.

In terms of traditional symbolism, caraway was considered a Herb of Consecration. This means that it was thought to possess the power to confer sanctity – when directed by intention and intuitive thought. By declaring something sacred, we transform our perception of it as something ephemeral into something eternal.

Caraway seeds were therefore added to wedding cakes to bless the union, and were distilled to provide an ingredient of medieval love potions, to encourage constancy and help ensure fidelity. In a similar way, it was thought that the seeds afforded the gift of retention, preventing the theft of any object that contained them.

Psychologically, caraway oil is particularly appropriate for individuals who were raised in unstable emotional environments. Though he or she may seek, as a sentimental ideal, the stability they were denied when young, the memories of a fluctuating childhood remain with them unconsciously, and find expression whenever emotional intimacy demands commitment. Their tendency is to shy away from such situations. They fear any form of stability they are unfamiliar with, doubting both its reality and their ability to be consistent.

Reinforcing the Earth Element, caraway restores our capacity to remain "centred" and steadfast. Its consolidates and "earths" a mercurial mind, and conveys a feeling of confidence. It is called for whenever a restless search for quick and easy solutions threatens to undermine our constancy and firm resolve.

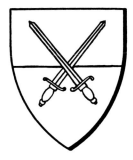

THE KNIGHT'S SWORD
Caraway seeds were used in an esoteric context to consecrate the knight's sword, itself a symbol of the straight and true, of conscious mastery over crude instinct.

Cardamom

appetite Ø stability Ø contentment

Cardamom is a reed-like perennial herb, growing to a height of three metres (nine feet), with oblong leaves, small yellow flowers with violet lips, and pale-yellow fruits containing reddish-brown ovoid seeds. It is the seeds that contain the essential oil. The plant is native to Sri Lanka and southern India, where it grows abundantly in humid forests and woody hillsides at heights of 750 to 1,500 metres (2,500 to 5,000 feet) above sea level.

For over 3,000 years, cardamom has been used extensively in both Chinese and Ayurvedic (traditional Indian) medicine. Imported to Greece from the 4th century BC, it was used by Greek physicians including Hippocrates, the father of Western medicine. The 17th-century English herbalist William Cole considered it the "chief of all seeds", writing that "it draweth forth flegmatick humours from both head and stomach".

The name *cardamom* is thought to have originated from the Arab, *hehmama,* a derivation of the Sanskrit term for something hot and pungent. The seeds have, in this regard, remained an important culinary spice in India, Europe, and the Middle East, where they are called "grains of paradise".

Traditionally, cardamom seeds have been used for a wide range of complaints including fluid retention, coughs, and various nervous disorders. In the East, they have also been valued as an aphrodisiac.

The therapeutic qualities of the oil are similar to those of caraway and fennel. While it is a general tonic of the body's vital energy, its principal use lies in the treatment of digestive complaints, especially those caused by stagnation of *Qi-energy* in the Stomach and intestines.

Stimulating the movement of digestive *Qi*, cardamom is carminative and antispasmodic: it helps to relieve indigestion and nausea, abdominal distention and colic, and hiccough and flatulence. The fact that the seeds are chewed to "sweeten the breath" – a common practice in India – demonstrates its value in neutralizing halitosis ("bad breath").

The generally fortifying influence of cardamom lies in its

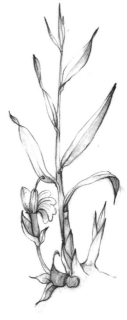

CARDAMOM
Elettaria cardamomum
FAMILY: *Zingiberaceae*
PARTS USED: *The seeds*
AROMA: *Warm, spicy, sweet, balsamic & slightly camphoraceous*
ENERGY: *Warm & dry*
MAIN ELEMENT: *Earth*
PROPERTIES: *Anticatarrhal, anti-infectious, antispasmodic, aperitive, calmative, carminative, digestive stimulant, expectorant, neurotonic, sexual tonic, sialogogic, stomachic, general tonic*
SAFETY DATA: *Non-toxic; non-irritant.*

ability to strengthen the *Qi-energy* of the Spleen-pancreas, the main organ responsible for transforming food and drink into *Qi* and *blood*. Whenever *Spleen-Qi* deficiency results in lethargy, poor appetite, and loose stools, the use of the oil may be considered.

Just as the warm sweetness of the oil's aroma reflects its action on the Spleen and Stomach, its pungent, slightly camphoraceous notes stimulate the *Qi-energy* of the Lungs. It is particularly helpful in cases where digestive weakness has lead to an accumulation of bronchial mucus, resulting in coughing and wheezing. Here, the oil acts as an expectorant and anticatarrhal.

Described as a cephalic, cardamom oil is also considered a gentle tonic of the brain and nervous system. Energetically, it supports the Spleen in its functions of housing the Intellect *(Yi)* and of raising *Qi* to the head. Like clary sage and marjoram oils, it can aid concentration if we are mentally sluggish, yet help to relax us when we are worried or tense. Together with other oils associated with the Earth Element, it is innately stabilizing and balancing.

Psychologically, therefore, cardamom oil is indicated for problems associated with the Earth Element: for poor concentration, overthinking, and worry – especially where there is a degree of nervous exhaustion. When burdened and weighed-down by worries, by responsibilities that test our endurance, the oil relaxes us, yet firms our resolve. At a more subtle level, we can think of the aphrodisiac and aperitive qualities of cardamom oil as helping to restore an "appetite for life". Whenever we feel deprived of opportunity or generosity, and fear that we may be denied fulfilment, cardamom oil reminds us of life's true abundance, and restores our desire for contentment.

Associated with Taurus, symbol of stability and appetite, it promotes a sense of earthy realism, helping us to assimilate the world as it is. At the same time, the oil is uplifting, and re-engages our hunger for life and its sustenance.

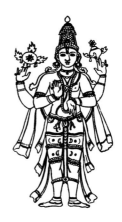

VISHNU, THE PRESERVER
Vishnu, the Hindu god referred to as the Preserver, reflects the supportive and sustaining qualities of cardamom oil. Vishnu's eighth incarnation is Krishna, whose love for the milkmaid Radha is seen as a deification of daily life.

Cedarwood

strength ◊ endurance ◊ certainty

Cedarwood oil is normally produced from the reddish-brown wood of the Atlas cedar tree, a large, spreading, evergreen conifer that grows to a height of 40 to 50 metres (135 to 165 feet). The leaves are needle-like and grey-green in colour, carried in clusters around the stems or branches; the brown cones are cylindrical and about eight centimetres (two inches) in length.

Atlas cedar *(Cedrus atlantica)* is native to the Atlas mountains of Algeria and Morocco, and is a close relative of the biblical cedar of Lebanon *(Cedrus libani)*. It should be distinguished from the North American Red cedar *(Juniperus virginiana)*, an entirely different genus that produces an essential oil of its own.

It was the original Lebanese cedar that for centuries was used to build temples, ships, and palaces throughout the Middle East. The wood was a popular building material because its high proportion of essential oil meant that it repelled both insects and fungus, and, like sandalwood, resisted decay. The Ancient Egyptians therefore used it to entomb their dead, and employed the oil in the mummification process. They valued it, too, as a ritual incense, cosmetic, and perfume.

Cedar appears repeatedly in the Bible, and according to the Song of Solomon was used to build Solomon's temple. It came to symbolize abundance, fertility, and spiritual strength; the name *cedrus* originating from the Arabic word *kedron*, meaning "power".

Indeed, cedarwood as an essential oil is fortifying and strengthening – a powerful tonic of the body's *Qi-energy*. Tonifying both the Kidneys and Spleen-pancreas, it may be used for general lethargy, nervous debility, lower backache, and poor concentration.

At the same time, cedarwood is a decongesting essential oil that encourages lymphatic drainage and stimulates the breakdown of accumulated fats. Mildly diuretic in action, it may be used for excessive weight gain, cellulite, and oedema (fluid retention). As an astringent remedy that helps to drain *cold*

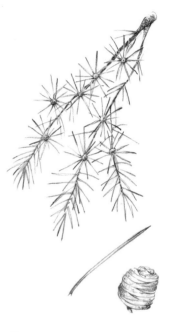

Cedarwood
Cedrus atlantica
Family: *Pinaceae*
Parts used: *The wood*
Aroma: *Woody, sweet, balsamic & slightly camphoraceous*
Energy: *Warm & dry*
Main element: *Water*
Properties: *Antibacterial, anticatarrhal, anti-infectious, antiseborrhoeic, arterial regenerator, astringent, calmative, cicatrisant, diuretic (mild), expectorant, lipolytic, lymphatic decongestant, general tonic*
Safety data: *Non-toxic; non-irritant*

dampness, it may also be used for abdominal distention with recurrent diarrhoea.

The decongesting nature of the oil combines with its anti-infectious properties to make it helpful for genito-urinary and respiratory infections – again, where the terrain, or underlying condition, is one of *cold dampness*. In cases of cystitis and urinary tract infection characterized by cramping pain, cedarwood oil may be combined with those of eucalyptus, thyme, and lavender, and applied as part of an ointment to the lower abdomen.

In terms of skin and hair care, cedarwood oil may be used for improving oily skin, acne, dandruff, and seborrhoea of the scalp.

Cedarwood oil's ability to strengthen the energetic function of the Kidneys relates psychologically to its fortifying action on the Will *(Zhi)*. In contrast to ginger, it does not stimulate the will-power *to action* so much as give us the will *to hold firm*, even against persistent external forces.

Cedarwood oil can therefore give us immovable strength in times of crisis. Steadying the conscious mind, it helps us to resist the sudden events and powerful emotions that threaten to undermine our confidence and morale. It can "buck-up" the ego when we feel alienated or destabilized – when we find ourselves, for example, suffering from "culture shock" in a foreign country or in a strange situation.

On a more subtle level, cedarwood oil can restore a sense of spiritual certainty similar in nature to caraway. While caraway oil reinforces the *unwavering determination* of the will – symbolized by the magical sword – cedarwood bolsters the *transforming power* of the will, and was used instead to consecrate the magical wand. The oil's deeply virile woody-balsamic aroma is one that helps us to take a negative or threatening situation, and transform it into an experience from which we can derive strength and wisdom.

WOTAN, THE FURY OF THE NIGHT
Cedar was used by the Nordic peoples to invoke the spirit of Wotan, either as a sacrificial incense or by using a staff or wand of the wood. The one-eyed god of storm, magic, and harvest, Wotan inspires our instinctual fortitude to weather turbulent circumstances, and make them, in the end, productive.

Chamomile

calm control ⌀ easy acceptance

Chamomile is the name given to several species of herbs with fine, almost feathery, leaves and daisy-like flowers. The two plants most commonly distilled for their essential oils are Roman, common, or noble chamomile *(Chamaemeleum nobile,* or *Anthemis nobilis)*, and German or wild chamomile *(Chamomilla recutita,* or *Matricaria chamomilla)*. The therapeutic and psychological properties of their respective oils, while not identical, are very similar.

Roman chamomile has been used for centuries in Europe as a medicine, fumigant, and ornamental flower. An important plant in Ancient Egypt, it was dedicated to Ra, the sun god, while in Greece, in the 4th century BC, it was employed by Hippocrates to help reduce fevers. In Tudor times in England chamomile was used as an aromatic strewing herb, trodden into household floors to delicately scent the home.

The name chamomile is derived from the Greek words *kamai* and *melon,* meaning "ground-apple", due to the apple-like scent of *Chamaemeleum nobile.* The Spanish word for chamomile, *manzanilla,* likewise means "little apple". *Matricaria,* on the other hand, comes from the Latin word *matrix,* meaning "womb", reflecting the herb's age-old use as a remedy for treating menstrual disorders.

In terms of Oriental medicine, the oils of both *Chamaemeleum nobile* and *Chamomilla recutita* have two main overall actions. The first is that of smoothing the flow of the body's *Qi-energy.* Chamomile oil's ability to regulate the movement of vital energy helps to relax the nerves, relieve spasm, and ease pain. This makes it beneficial for chronic tension and insomnia; nervous indigestion and nausea; constipation and irritable bowel; headache and asthma. Combined with cypress and clary sage oils, it is also useful for relieving both premenstrual tension and menstrual pain. Of the two varieties, it is *Chamaemeleum nobile* that excels as an antispasmodic, analgesic, and carminative essential oil.

The second overall action of the chamomile oils – and one that adds to their well-known calmative effect – is that of clearing *heat* and reducing inflammation. It is this general

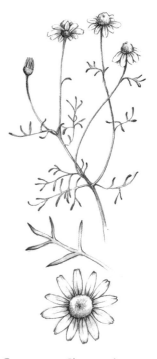

CHAMOMILE *Chamaemeleum nobile & Chamomilla recutita*
FAMILY: *Compositae (Asteraceae)*
PARTS USED: *The flowering head*
AROMA: *Roman chamomile (Chamaemeleum nobile) is sweet, warm, herbaceous & slightly fruity; German chamomile (Chamomilla recutita), while sweet & hay-like, is more bitter*
ENERGY: *Cool/ neutral moisture*
MAIN ELEMENT: *Wood*
PROPERTIES: *Analgesic, anti-allergenic, anti-inflammatory, antineuralgic, antiparasitic, antispasmodic, calmative, carminative, digestive stimulant, ophthalmic, stomachic*
SAFETY DATA: *Non-toxic; non-irritant*

property that makes *Chamomilla recutita*, in particular, helpful for alleviating gastritis, neuritis, cystitis, rheumatoid arthritis, and earache. One of the most important essential oils for the skin, German chamomile may be combined with lavender and geranium oils in the treatment of dermatitis, eczema, and pruritus (itching).

The key to understanding the psychological effect of chamomile lies in grasping its energetic influence on the solar plexus – the major nerve centre located in the stomach area. Lying half-way between the region of "gut instinct" and that of the empathetic heart, the solar plexus is the vital centre of our psychological needs and wants. It is the focus both of our urge to control and desire to nurture, and of our search for recognition and sense of self-worth. In keeping with the function of the Wood Element, the solar plexus channels the drives of the ego, guiding them toward self-fulfilment through the power of self-control.

Chamomile oil can help to relieve nervous stress of any kind, but is of greatest benefit for problems associated with a build-up of tension in the solar plexus. When in this condition, our emotional needs and wants have usually intensified, and if they are frustrated, we can become vexed and irritable. We may react by trying even harder to achieve or grasp them – by "over-controlling" to the point where we may "lose control". We then criticize ourselves for being weak and childish, or moodily blame others from whom we expected more.

Chamomile eases the tension of excessive ego-desire – and the frustration, resentment, and depression that frequently follow. Its warm, apple-like fragrance imparts a sense of satisfaction, while its gentle bitterness cools us with a taste of reality. The chamomiles help us to let go of fixed expectations, calmly acknowledge our own limitations, and more readily accept the help and support that others can manage to give. A more "sunny" disposition will always emerge.

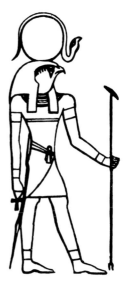

RA, THE EGYPTIAN SUN GOD
Chamomile was used to invoke solar deities such as the Egyptian sun god Ra (or "creator"). An important remedy in Ancient Egyptian medicine, chamomile is an emblem of the omnipotence of Ra through its power to restore wholeness to the Self.

Clary Sage

revitalize ∅ clarify ∅ inspire

Clary sage is a biennial or perennial herb, growing 30 to 120 centimetres (11 inches to four feet) high, with hairy heart-shaped leaves and numerous pale-blue, lavender-pink or white flowers. The plant belongs to a genus that consists of some 450 species of hardy evergreen subshrubs, all native to southern Europe. Clary sage can be found throughout the European continent, growing wild and cultivated in gardens.

The English name *clary* is derived from the Latin word *clarus*, meaning "clear" – reflecting the role of the plant in the treatment of eye complaints. A traditional herbal infusion was made from the seeds and applied to strained or sore eyes. The name of the genus, *Salvia*, is derived from the Latin word *salvere*, meaning "to save, or heal". This reflected the immense reputation of common sage as a curative plant which ensured longevity, the reason it was called *herba sacra*, or "sacred herb", by the Romans.

The essential oil of common sage *(Salvia officinalis)* does, however, have an important limitation. The fact that it is composed of up to 50% thujone, a potentially toxic ketone, renders it unsuitable for normal usage. However, essential oil of clary sage *(Salvia sclarea)* is completely safe in normal doses, and is one of the most important aromatics used in aromatherapy.

This stems in part from its ability, like marjoram oil, to calm states of tension, yet revive those of fatigue. In terms of Oriental medicine, clary sage oil both strengthens *Qi-energy* that is depleted, and relaxes and circulates *Qi-energy* that is "stuck". Hence, it is both an effective general tonic and major antispasmodic.

In terms of its regulating, antispasmodic, analgesic action, clary sage is indicated, like lavender oil, for muscular stiffness and spasm, tired, aching legs, headache, and migraine. Smoothing the flow of *Qi-energy* in the Stomach and intestines, it can in addition relieve abdominal distention, flatulence, and symptoms of irritable bowel. A gynaecological remedy of equal importance to cypress, the oil may be used to reduce premenstrual tension, and to help ease menstrual

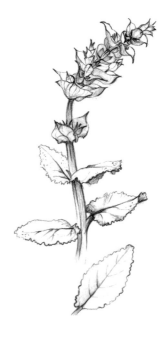

CLARY SAGE
Salvia sclarea
FAMILY: *Labiatae (Lamiaceae)*
PARTS USED: *The flowering tops and leaves*
AROMA: *Warm, camphoraceous, bittersweet, musky & slightly spicy*
ENERGY: *Neutral temperature/ dry*
MAIN ELEMENT: *Metal*
PROPERTIES: *Antibacterial, anti-depressive, antifungal, anti-infectious, antispasmodic, astringent, carminative, digestive stimulant, neurotonic, phlebotonic, stomachic, uterine tonic*
SAFETY DATA: *Non-toxic; non-irritant*

pain. It is also useful to dull pain during labour.

The benefits of clary sage oil to the respiratory system clearly demonstrate the versatility of its actions. It can be used to both strengthen *and* circulate *Lung-Qi*, and is therefore indicated for fatigue and shallow breathing on the one hand, and asthmatic symptoms on the other. Helping to deepen the breath, clary sage works to "open the chest" when it feels stuffy, tight, or constricted. As a mildly expectorant, anti-infectious essential oil, it may in addition be combined with those of eucalyptus and pine for catarrhal coughs, throat infections, and bronchitis.

The psychological actions of clary sage oil are closely linked to its energetic ones, and the balance it creates between stimulation and relaxation. A general and neuro-tonic indicated for mental fatigue and nervous debility, the oil is, on the other hand, effective for calming the mind and easing tension. Strengthening yet relaxing, the net effect of clary sage oil is one of mental-emotional uplift, and of the euphoria for which the oil is renowned.

However, the type of uplift that clary sage oil promotes is not one that is "ungrounded" or disconnected from reality. The earthy quality of its herbaceous, musky sweetness reflects its ability to both steady the mind and reassure; while its gentle pungency enlivens the senses and dispels illusion, restoring the clarity echoed by its name. The oil is therefore indicated, in particular, for nervous anxiety and depression characterized by changeable moods, indecision, and emo-tional confusion.

With a pronounced effect on both the Lungs and the *Qi-energy*, clary sage acts strongly on the Bodily Soul *(P'o)*. When the Bodily Soul is afflicted by despondency or worry, we can lose a "felt instinct" for our life's true purpose, unable to "see" clearly in the here and now. Absorbed by the deliber-ations of a restless, searching mind, we are distracted from the Spirit and its intuitive insight. Through releasing con-striction within the vital body, and restoring lucidity to the instincts, clary sage oil allows inspiration to flow.

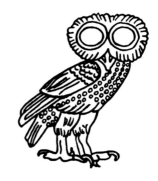

THE OWL OF WISDOM
Although a symbol of death in Celtic, Christian, Egyptian, and Chinese mythology, the owl to the Greeks, Romans, and native Americans represented wisdom. Clary sage imbues sagacity and insight, and helps us to come to terms with loss .

Coriander

joyful stability ∅ calm creativity

Coriander is a hardy annual herb, growing 30-90 centimetres (11 to 33 inches) high, with delicate bright-green leaves, umbels of dainty white flowers, and bunches of small round fruits that turn from green to brown as they ripen. Native to the Mediterranean and western Asia, coriander is cultivated commercially throughout the world, and in temperate regions is a widespread weed. The seed as well as the leaf of the plant yields an essential oil, the oil from the seed being produced in Russia, Romania, and Vietnam.

The name *coriandrum* is derived from the Latin *koros*, meaning "bed-bug". This is because the stinking odour of its fresh leaves apparently resembled the insect's smell.

Coriander seeds have been a popular aromatic stimulant and culinary spice since time immemorial. Cultivated for over 3,000 years, coriander is mentioned in all the medieval medical texts, by the Greeks, in the Bible, and by early Sanskrit writers. Appearing in the Ebers papyrus, the Ancient Egyptians steeped coriander and fresh garlic in wine, and drank it as an aphrodisiac. Believing it to contain the secret of happiness, it was among the plants offered to the temple gods, the seeds having been found at the tombs of both Tutankhamun and Rameses II.

Indigenous to the Holy Land, coriander was compared by the Ancient Hebrews to the *manna* provided by God to the Children of Israel, and was one of the bitter herbs eaten at the Passover. Featuring in traditional Chinese medicine as a tonic of the Stomach and Heart, the herb in Ancient China was thought to promote longevity and to ease pain.

In medieval Europe, coriander was considered to be an aphrodisiac – and a witch's herb employed in love magic and love potions. In Tudor times in England it was an ingredient of the popular drink "Hippocras", offered to guests to raise their spirits at weddings and festive occasions.

From an energetic perspective, coriander is *warm* and *dry* in nature, and shares the same digestive, carminative proper-ties as other essential oils distilled from *Umbelliferae* plants; caraway and fennel included.

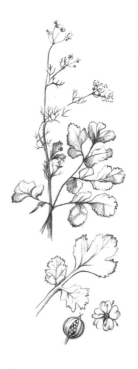

CORIANDER
Coriandrum sativum
FAMILY: *Umbelliferae (Apiaceae)*
PART USED: *The crushed ripe seeds*
AROMA: *Warm, spicy, woody, sweet & slightly camphoraceous*
ENERGY: *Warm & dry*
MAIN ELEMENT: *Earth (& Fire)*
PROPERTIES: *Analgesic, anti-bacterial, antidepressive, anti-infectious, antispasmodic, aperitive, carminative, digestive stimulant, neurotonic, stomachic, general tonic*
SAFETY DATA: *Non-toxic; non-irritant*

Circulating *Qi-energy* in the Stomach and intestines, coriander seed oil is an excellent digestive antispasmodic, useful for poor appetite, indigestion, abdominal distention, and flatulence.

It can also be used to circulate the *Qi* and disperse *cold* in cases of *painful obstruction* – the energetic condition used to describe osteoarthritis, neuralgia, and rheumatic pain. Combined with oils of marjoram and clary sage, it may be used, in addition, to alleviate muscular pain and stiffness.

Like cardamom, coriander seed oil strengthens the function of the Spleen-pancreas and Stomach, and therefore invigorates the Intellect *(Yi)*. This accounts in part for its neurotonic property. Fortifying both the *Qi* and the nerves, the oil is indicated for general debility, mental fatigue, and nervous exhaustion.

Coriander's action on the Spleen, Stomach, and Intellect *(Yi)* associate it psychologically with the Element Earth. At the same time, its spicy, slightly musky aroma, and its reputation as a euphoric and aphrodisiac link it to the Element Fire. Combining a warm and woody serenity with peppery stimulation, the oil both calms and uplifts, and is indicated, therefore, for states of nervous depression that are accompanied by worry and anxious overthinking. Coriander is consequently symbolized by both the stimulating Mars and comforting Moon.

Traditionally classified as a Herb of Protection and of Immortality, coriander, like caraway, imbues a feeling of security, peace, and earthy permanence. Yet it couples this with a feeling of spontaneity and passion, and seeks to achieve stability without denying joy.

Coriander seed oil is ideally suited, therefore, to complex, creative individuals who find it difficult to cope with predictability and routine. Although they need stability and emotional security, the resilience they seek is borne of passionate involvement, rather than of self-protection.

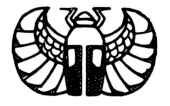

THE EGYPTIAN SCARABAEUS
The great scarab beetle pushed the fiery ball of the sun along its path across the sky. An Egyptian symbol of fertility, virility, and divine wisdom, it mirrors both the aphrodisiac and inspirational qualities of coriander seed oil.

Cypress

transition ∅ transformation ∅ renewal

Cypress is an evergreen conifer that grows to a height of 25-45 metres (82 to 147 feet). Although it bears small flowers that produce round greyish-brown cones, it is the fresh dark-green leaves and twigs that contain most of the essential oil. According to Ernest Guenther, "it is a tree of serene beauty, blending well into the Mediterranean landscape; its dark foliage contrasts with the lucid sky, and etches delicate silhouettes against the blue sea". Native to southern Europe, Italian cypress *(Cupressus sempervirens)* has spread to North Africa and North America, and is cultivated in France, Spain, and Morocco.

The use of cypress as an incense and medicine was first recorded in the papyri of Ancient Egypt, where it was employed to make sarcophagi. The Ancient Greeks dedicated the tree to Hades (or Pluto), god of the Underworld, associating it with death and eternity. It was for this reason planted in graveyards throughout the Mediterranean, as a symbol of grief and as a source of solace. This was a practice that continued for centuries.

Both the leaves and cones of cypress have long been valued for their astringent (or binding) action. In fact, the leaves were first used for curing haemorrhoids by the Ancient Assyrians, while the Greek physician Galen (AD 165) recommended them for internal bleeding and diarrhoea. Cypress has an equally ancient reputation for alleviating menstrual disorders.

In terms of Oriental medicine, the principal action of cypress oil is to enliven and regulate the flow of *blood*. Part of this action depends upon its restorative, toning effect on the veins, a by-product of its overall astringent quality. The oil may be combined with those of clary sage, lemon, and geranium, and applied as an ointment for haemorrhoids and varicose veins.

Cypress oil's *cool*, astringent nature also helps to reduce excessive perspiration, making it a useful and effective deodorant for sweaty feet.

The ability of cypress oil to harmonize the flow of *blood* also makes it important for menstrual problems. It is one of

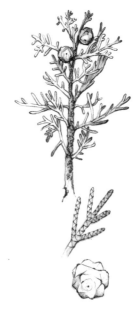

CYPRESS
Cupressus sempervirens var. stricta
FAMILY: *Cupressaceae*
PARTS USED: *The fresh leaves and twigs*
AROMA: *Fresh, piney, balsamic, sweet & slightly citrus*
ENERGY: *Cool & dry*
MAIN ELEMENT: *Metal (& Water)*
PROPERTIES: *Antibacterial, anti-infectious, antirheumatic, antispasmodic, antisudorific, astringent, calmative, deodorant, diuretic (mild), lymphatic decongestant, neurotonic, phlebotonic, prostatic decongestant*
SAFETY DATA: *Non-toxic; non-irritant*

the main essential oils for both dysmenorrhoea (menstrual pain) and menorrhagia (excessive menstrual bleeding).

Cypress oil not only moves the *blood*, but helps, in addition, to circulate *Qi-energy*. Like lavender and other oils, this action provides it with a wide-ranging antispasmodic potential, of benefit for spasmodic colitis, premenstrual tension, and asthma. A generally decongesting, detoxifying essential oil, it may also be used for acne, skin rashes, lymphatic congestion, and rheumatic pain.

Cypress oil has one of the most distinct and profound of psychological actions. The sour, astringent, and woody notes of the essence convey a feeling of cohesion and stability. At the same time, its fresh, coniferous pungency, and ability to circulate the *Qi* and *blood*, relate it to both psychological transition and real-life change. Cypress oil's basic subtle action, then, is to help us cope with and accept even difficult change – of both an inner and outer nature.

Through encouraging the process of "taking in and letting go" – of the ability to accept and relinquish – cypress reinforces the Bodily Soul *(P'o)*, the vital spirit of the Lungs. Dissolving remorse and instilling optimism, cypress oil helps us to flow with the flux of life. From here we can contemplate the tree's long and deep relationship to death and the grieving process, and why it was thought to be of comfort to those in bereavement.

That cypress has been dedicated to Pluto – a symbol in astrology of psychological transformation – further reinforcing its connection to inner renewal. The oil's association with Pluto reflects the potential it has to unearth the fears that block change. The oil may therefore be considered for states of mind characterized by a conscious urge to find a new direction, yet one frustrated by an equally powerful, often hidden, sense of self-doubt. Strengthening our capacity to both channel and contain, cypress allows suppressed, obstructive feelings to emerge to consciousness, liberating the energy that we spend in keeping them locked within.

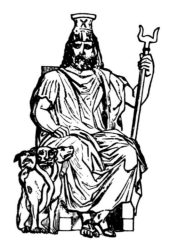

HADES, LORD OF THE UNDERWORLD
Cypress was dedicated to Hades (the "unseen"), the Greek god of death whose Roman equivalent is Pluto. Its serenely supportive fragrance possesses the power to both comfort grief and abate the fears that lurk in the "underworld" of the psyche.

Eucalyptus

optimism ∅ openness ∅ freedom

Eucalyptus is an evergreen tree that grows to a height of 100 metres (328 feet), making it one of the world's tallest trees. It has leathery lanceolate leaves of a pale blue-green colour, and small white flowers, which, in bud, are covered by a cap-like membrane. It is the presence of this "lid" which has led to the tree's common name, derived from the Greek *eucalyptos*, meaning "well-covered". Native to Australia and Tasmania, the tree today grows the world over, China being the largest exporter of the essential oil.

There are over 700 varieties of eucalyptus, of which more than 500 produce an essential oil! In addition to *Eucalyptus globulus*, other species commonly distilled for their essence include: narrow-leaved eucalyptus *(Euc. radiata)* – useful for viral infections; lemon-scented eucalyptus *(Euc. citriadora)* – a cooling antirheumatic; and peppermint-scented eucalyptus *(Euc. dives piperitoniferum)* – good for mucous colitis. Eucalyptus oil shares many of the same actions as those of tea tree, myrtle, cajuput, and niaouli – all members of the *Myrtaceae* family.

Eucalyptus was first employed medicinally by the aboriginal peoples of Australia, who used it to treat infections and fevers, especially as a fumigant. Following its discovery by the French naturalist De Labillardiere, "Fever Tree", as it became known, was planted in some of the most marshy and malarial regions of Algiers, due to the powerful drying action of the roots on the soil. While the strongly anti-infectious oil was inhaled to reduce malarial fever, the tree transformed some of the most marshy areas into the driest.

A major expectorant and anticatarrhal essential oil, eucalyptus's principal sphere of action is on the respiratory system. Here, its pungent, camphoraceous aroma can be seen at work through its unparalleled ability to clear *Lung-phlegm*. Its antibacterial, antiviral action makes it useful, in addition, for the common cold, sinusitis, laryngitis, and chronic bronchitis. A tonic of the *Lung-Qi*, eucalyptus oil generally enhances the breathing function, promoting the uptake of oxygen by the red blood cells.

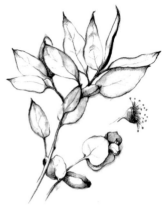

EUCALYPTUS
Eucalyptus globulus
FAMILY: *Myrtaceae*
PARTS USED: *The leaf*
AROMA: *Strong, fresh, camphoraceous, balsamic & slightly sweet*
ENERGY: *Warm & dry*
MAIN ELEMENT: *Metal*
PROPERTIES: *Antibacterial, anticatarrhal, antifungal, anti-infectious, antirheumatic, antiviral, balsamic, decongestant, diuretic (mild), expectorant, febrifuge, hypoglycaemic, immune tonic, insect repellent, rubefacient*
SAFETY DATA: *Non-toxic; non-irritant*

The germicidal action of eucalyptus oil extends to the genito-urinary system, where it is indicated for cystitis and leucorrhoea. Its value in such conditions is enhanced by its ability to clear the *dampness* or congestive *terrain*, which, by providing a breeding ground for microbes, makes infection more likely. The oil is, in this and other ways, an immune tonic, and may be combined with oils of tea tree and common thyme to strengthen the *Defensive-Qi* and prevent infection from recurring.

The stimulating, decongesting and balsamic (soothing) qualities of the essential oil make it further indicated for rheumatic pain of a *cold*, cramping nature. It may also be applied to relieve muscular pain and neuralgia.

The psychological properties of *Eucalyptus globulus* – and the genus as a whole – are closely related to its energetic action on the Lungs. As the oil improves breathing, and decongests and "opens the chest", it is of direct benefit to the Bodily Soul *(P'o)*. Its fresh, pungent, yet soothing aroma helps to dispel melancholy and revive the spirits, working to restore both vitality and a positive outlook.

At a deeper level, the essence of this tall and swamp-draining tree can help promote within us a wider perspective on life. Penetrating and cleansing, it dispels the half-conscious, stagnated feelings that can keep us bound to a limiting environment.

Eucalyptus oil is suited to people who feel emotionally "hemmed-in" or constricted by their surroundings – whether at home, at work, or in society. They sense the possibility of achieving greater freedom and a wider life experience, but dare not seek to create this due to excessive caution, habit, fear, or responsibility. Eucalyptus oil helps to disperse the negative feelings associated with such situations, and gives us, inwardly, "room to breathe". Whether the inspiration it instills leads to change or greater acceptance, the oil can transform a sense of suffocation into one of expansive renewal.

THE FREEDOM OF THE HUNTER
This representation of a hunter made by Bushmen of the Kalahari evokes the vital, free-spirited sense of adventure inspired by oil of eucalyptus.

Everlasting

unblock Ø relinquish Ø forgive

Everlasting is an aromatic shrub, growing to a height of 60 centimetres (22 inches), with silvery-grey lanceolate leaves and clusters of small bright-yellow flowers. When dried, the plant keeps its shape and the flower-heads their yellow colour – hence they are "everlasting". Native to the Mediterranean basin, the plant grows in Dalmatia, Italy, France, and Spain.

Also known as "immortelle" and "Italian straw flower", everlasting was traditionally used in Europe for scrofula, asthma, arthritis, and headaches. The herb was also taken to help expel worms. In homeopathy, a tincture is prepared from the fresh plant and prescribed for gall bladder disorders and lumbago.

The medicinal and psychological actions of everlasting oil make it unique, and one of the most powerful of aromatic essences. It is somewhat similar in its properties to Roman chamomile and yarrow, sibling members of the *Compositae* family. All three essential oils regulate the flow of *Qi-energy*, encourage the flow of bile and have an important anti-spasmodic effect. They also share an ability to clear *heat* and reduce inflammation. Everlasting oil does, however, have therapeutic characteristics that are quite distinct.

In terms of problems that relate to a stagnation of *Qi-energy*, the oil is indicated for headache and migraine, muscular aches and pains, neuralgia, and irritable bowel. As its strongly antispasmodic property is coupled with an anticatarrhal action, the oil can also benefit chronic coughs and asthma.

What makes everlasting oil unique is its ability to regulate not only the *Qi*, but the *blood* as well. Among its chemical constituents are a group of ketone-like compounds called beta-diones. It is this group of molecules within the oil that contribute in the main to its anticoagulant action, making it applicable in the treatment of any severe bruising that results in haematoma (accumulated, clotted blood). When combined with the oil's anti-inflammatory influence on the veins, this property extends to making it helpful in cases of thrombophlebitis, where inflammation and degeneration of the veins lead to clot formation.

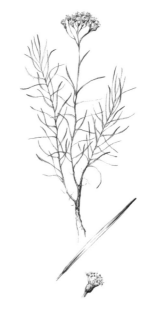

EVERLASTING (IMMORTELLE)
Helichrysum italicum ssp. serotinum
FAMILY: *Compositae (Asteraceae)*
PARTS USED: *The flowering head*
AROMA: *Bittersweet, warm, rich & curry-like*
ENERGY: *Cool & dry*
MAIN ELEMENT: *Wood*
PROPERTIES: *Anti-allergenic, anticatarrhal, anticoagulant, anti-haematomic, anti-inflammatory, antispasmodic, calmative, cholagogic, cicatrisant, expectorant, hepatic stimulant*
SAFETY DATA: *Non-toxic; non-irritant*

The anti-inflammatory, decongesting actions of everlasting oil are useful in conditions of bronchitis, colitis, and rheumatoid arthritis. In common with German chamomile oil, it is also effective for allergic conditions, particularly those which involve nasal catarrh, sneezing, and itchy skin rashes.

Everlasting oil's ability to move stagnant *Qi-energy* and *blood* relate it, via the Liver, to the Wood Element and the Ethereal Soul *(Hun)*. Sharing with chamomile a warm bittersweet aroma, it has a parallel psychological effect on the irritable, moody states that we can associate with stagnant *Qi*. Both everlasting and chamomile relax and comfort the solar plexus area, alleviating the tension that arises from over-effort and over-control, and the depression generated from long-standing frustration.

Where everlasting oil departs from the more gentle, soothing chamomile is in its rich curry-like pungency and ability to disperse more deeply embedded repression. Everlasting oil's capacity to dissolve clots and regulate *stagnant blood* – conditions associated with the Liver – gives it, on a subtle level, the power to break through the deepest, most "stuck" of negative emotions. Those specifically indicated are linked to the Wood Element: enduring resentment, half-conscious anger, bitterness of spirit, and a stubbornly negative attitude.

Such individuals are emotionally "blocked" in a profound way, unable not only to give expression to their anger and despair but to admit to themselves the fact of their own deep wounding. Instead of seeking ways to release these feelings – feelings which may stem from childhood emotional trauma – they respond instead by developing rigid, self-denying thought patterns, and by judging harshly those who are open and spontaneous. Though secretly despairing, they cannot bear to see others admit vulnerability, and may feel rage when they do so.

At its most transformative, everlasting oil can loosen the very hardest of knots lying deep within the psyche, restoring to the Ethereal Soul *(Hun)* its ultimate capacity for compassion – not only for others but first and foremost for oneself.

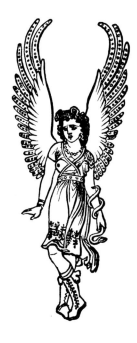

MEGAIRA, THE RESENTFUL ONE
One of the three avenging Furies of Greek mythology, Megaira is pictured here at her most benign. She symbolizes, from one perspective, the forces that can retard emotional and spiritual development – and the kind of smouldering fury that calls for everlasting oil.

$\mathcal{F}$ennel

self-expression Ø productivity Ø communication

Fennel is a hardy biennial or perennial herb, growing to a height of two metres (six feet), with fine, feathery leaves and umbels of golden-yellow flowers. The essential oil is produced from the crushed seeds. Indigenous to the shores of the Mediterranean, the plant now grows throughout Europe and in India, Japan, and North America.

There are two varieties of fennel: bitter or common fennel *(Foeniculum vulgare var. amara)* and sweet or garden fennel *(Foeniculum vulgare var. dulce)*. Sweet fennel is the preferred oil for use in aromatherapy, due to its more gentle nature and the lower proportion of fenchone it contains.

The use of fennel as a herb stretches back to antiquity, featuring in the culinary and medical arts of Ancient Egypt, Greece, Rome, and India, as well as in Anglo-Saxon cookery. The Greeks were among the first to recognize its value as a gently diuretic slimming aid, naming the herb *Marathron,* from *maraino,* to "grow thin". With an equal reputation for promoting strength and longevity, the seeds were eaten by athletes while training for the Olympic games. The Romans ate them as part of an after-meal seed cake to aid digestion, renaming the plant *foeniculum* – meaning "hay-like" – because of its sweet, dried-grass aroma. Traditionally classified as *warm* and *dry* in nature, fennel has long been valued for its carminative, diuretic, and tonic properties. It was, for centuries, also considered to improve eyesight and hearing.

Like caraway and cardamom, fennel's principal sphere of action is on the digestive system, where both the essential oil and herbal infusion stimulate the flow of *Qi-energy* in the Stomach and intestines. An effective antispasmodic of gastric and intestinal smooth muscle, the oil is used to relieve indigestion, abdominal bloating, nausea, belching, and flatulence. It may also be used to help "move the bowel" in cases of constipation.

Fennel oil's regulating action on the *Qi-energy* extends to the chest region. Together with its ability to disperse *cold phlegm*, it is a supportive remedy for both catarrhal coughs and nervous asthma.

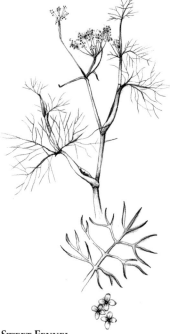

SWEET FENNEL
Foeniculum vulgare var. dulce
FAMILY: *Umbelliferae (Apiaceae)*
PARTS USED: *The seeds*
AROMA: *Sweet, pungent, anise-like*
ENERGY: *Warm & dry*
MAIN ELEMENT: *Earth*
PROPERTIES: *Analgesic, anti-infectious, antispasmodic, aperitive, carminative, cholagogic, digestive stimulant, diuretic, emmenagogic, expectorant, lactogenic, oestrogen-like, stomachic*
SAFETY DATA: *Do not use in pregnancy or while breast-feeding, or on children under 2 yrs. Avoid using on hypersensitive, diseased, or damaged skin and on those with endometriosis or oestrogen-dependent cancer. Do not use at more than 1% dilution.*

Invigorating *Qi-energy* in the Kidneys and Spleen, fennel is a mild diuretic and lymphatic decongestant, helping to rid the body of stagnant fluids and fats. A traditional slimming aid, fennel may be used for water retention, cellulite, and obesity, both as an essential oil and herbal tea.

The 17-century herbalist-astrologer Nicholas Culpeper associated fennel with the astrological planet Mercury and the sign of Virgo. While Virgo is linked to the intestines and to all that is practical and productive, Mercury is the archetypal symbol of the conscious, rational mind, and of communication.

We can make similar associations from the viewpoint of Oriental medicine. Fennel oil's warm, sweet aroma, together with its actions as an aperitive and digestive stimulant, relate it closely to the Earth Element and the Intellect *(Yi)*. An important aspect of the Earth Element is the need and capacity to be productive and creative.

Fennel is suited to the type of individual who tends to overthink and over-analyse. While they may easily generate concepts and ideas, they rarely communicate them or put them into practice. Finding it difficult to articulate and express themselves, feelings, too, tend to churn within. The more such emotions are locked inside, the more they intensify, building up tension that affects the bowels. The unacceptable, unexpressed thoughts and emotions that are pushed below consciousness accumulate in the intestines as nervous spasm and gas.

Fennel encourages us to express ourselves through the mouth rather than through the bottom! Freeing the feelings that have stagnated and putrefied, clearing the plethora of a congested mind, the oil invites us to communicate freely, without fear or inhibition.

By unblocking our capacity for confident self-expression, fennel oil releases our urge to create. It helps us to find, like oil of ginger, productive outlets for the active mind.

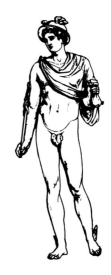

MERCURY, THE MESSENGER GOD
Fennel, like many of the Umbelliferae plants, has been linked to Mercury, the Roman equivalent of the Greek god Hermes. The light-footed messenger of the gods, Mercury is symbolic of our ability to express and communicate ourselves.

Frankincense

tranquil contemplation & spiritual liberation

Frankincense, or olibanum, is a small tree, which, growing to a height of three to seven metres (nine to 22 feet), has abundant narrow leaves and white or pale-pink flowers. Incisions are made into the trunk in order to allow a milky-white *oleo-resin* to exude. The resin then hardens into an orange-brown gum, and is steam-distilled for its essential oil. Native to the Middle East and North Africa, the tree grows in Somalia, Ethiopia, southern Arabia, and China.

Frankincense played a role in the religious and domestic life of the Ancient Egyptian, Babylonian, Persian, Hebrew, Greek, and Roman civilizations. It has been perhaps the most important aromatic incense ingredient since history began. This is reflected in the fact that its English name is derived from the medieval French word *franc*, meaning "pure" or "free", and the Latin *incensium*, "to smoke".

Employed by the Egyptians as a fumigant, ritual incense and cosmetic, frankincense gum was charred to produce a black powder called *kohl*, used by Egyptian women to paint their eyelids. It was in addition one of the main ingredients of *kyphi*, the renowned temple incense burned at sunset.

Frankincense is one of the four main ingredients that make up Jewish ceremonial incense, and has for centuries formed an integral part of the Sabbath day offering. Presented as a gift to the newly born Jesus, the gum is mentioned a total of 22 times in the Bible.

Frankincense oil's most important sphere of action must be the nervous system. Here, its ability to relax and yet revitalize make it excellent for treating both nervous tension and nervous exhaustion. It smooths the flow of stagnant *Qi-energy* whenever an accumulation of stress has led to irritability, restlessness, and insomnia. As a mild tonic, it can also help to uplift, and so is an important antidepressive essential oil.

The fact that frankincense oil possesses anticatarrhal and expectorant properties also makes it useful for bronchitis and asthma, especially when associated with nervous tension. The oil is said to "deepen the breath", and can help to relieve "tightness" in the chest. Anti-infectious and soothing, it may

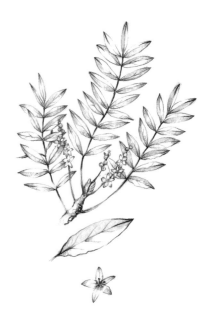

FRANKINCENSE
Boswellia carterii
FAMILY: *Burseraceae*
PARTS USED: *The gum*
AROMA: *Resinous, balsamic, rich, camphoraceous & slightly citrus*
ENERGY: *Cool & dry*
MAIN ELEMENT: *Earth (& Metal)*
PROPERTIES: *Analgesic, antibacterial, anticatarrhal, antidepressive, anti-infectious, astringent, balsamic, calmative, carminative, cicatrisant, expectorant, immune tonic, stomachic, vulnerary*
SAFETY DATA: *Non-toxic; non-irritant*

also be used for both sinusitis and laryngitis.

Frankincense oil's ability to smooth the flow of *Qi-energy* and calm the nerves means that, like essential oils of chamomile and lavender, it has a useful analgesic (pain-relieving) action. This is applicable for rheumatic, menstrual, and epigastric pain. Considered by some to strengthen the immune system, it is especially useful, like tea tree oil, in cases where nervous depression is in danger of weakening the *Defensive-Qi.*

Frankincense oil has profound psychological and spiritual benefits, long recognized by religious and spiritual traditions the world over. In terms of the Five Elements (see pp.30-45), the effect of frankincense oil may be linked on a fundamental level to that of Earth, where its ability to calm and centre the mind reflects its gently tranquillizing, yet deeply clarifying, effect on the Intellect *(Yi)*. Like sandalwood oil, it is an ideal aid to meditation, contemplation, and prayer, ceasing mental chatter and stilling the mind. Facilitating a state of single-pointed concentration, it allows the Spirit to soar.

On a day-to-day level, it may be called upon for states of mental agitation and worry, or whenever the mind is distract-ed and overwhelmed by a cacophony of thoughts.

Dedicated through the ages to a variety of solar deities – the Babylonian sun god Bael, the Egyptian god Ra and the Greek Apollo – frankincense contains the power to focus our spiritual consciousness, and imbue a potential for transcen-dent awareness. Whenever we have allowed ourselves to become oppressed by the mundane or tied to the past – indeed, restricted or weighed-down by any form of over-attachment – frankincense can help us to break free. This it will achieve through encouraging tranquillity, insight, and spiritual self-discipline, allowing the ego-self and trans-personal Self to work in unison.

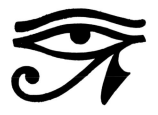

THE UTCHAT, OR SACRED EYE
Frankincense, like chamomile, was employed in the worship of the Egyptian sun god Ra, a primordial symbol for whom was the Utchat, or "All-seeing" – the sacred eye that burned with judgment. Frankincense oil rekindles the inner light of the mind.

Geranium

security ∅ receptivity ∅ intimacy

Geranium is a bushy perennial shrub, growing to a height of one metre (three feet), with hairy, serrated, heart-shaped leaves and dense umbels of pink flowers. The *Pelargonium* genus is a very extensive one, and includes over 200 different species, most of which originate from South Africa. Among the small number of species cultivated for their oil, it is the *Pelargonium graveolens* of the Réunion Islands which is thought to produce oil of the highest quality.

The name *Pelargonium* is derived from the Greek word *palargos*, or stork, since the fruit is thought to resemble a stork's bill.

There is very little historical reference to the *Pelargonium* genus. Introduced into Europe in the late 17th century, geranium became a popular garden plant, found today in most frost-free areas. It was the French chemist Recluz who in 1819 was the first to distil the leaves of geranium. It has since become an important perfume ingredient, and is often used as a substitute for oil of rose. The Italian doctor Rovesti employed geranium oil in the treatment of anxiety states.

Geranium is one of the few essential oils, which, in terms of Oriental medicine, may be considered *cool* and *moist* in energy. The oil clears *heat* and inflammation, relaxes the nerves, and calms feelings of anxiety. It also has the ability to strengthen *Qi-energy*.

As an anti-inflammatory essential oil, geranium may be compared to those of lavender and German chamomile, and is indicated for gastritis, colitis, psoriasis, and eczema. It can also be used for skin infections such as acne, impetigo, and athlete's foot.

Encouraging the circulation of *Qi* and *blood*, geranium oil is both analgesic and antispasmodic. It is particularly useful for nerve, eye, and joint pain, and is applicable in cases of neuralgia, ophthalmia, and rheumatism. Astringent and phlebotonic, the oil can also relieve haemorrhoids, varicose veins, and excessive menstrual bleeding.

As a tonic, geranium oil is able to reinforce both the *Qi-energy* of the Spleen and pancreas, and the *yin-energy* of the

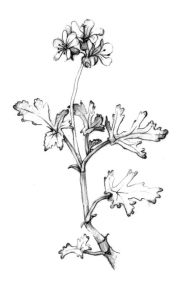

GERANIUM
Pelargonium x asperum/ graveolens
FAMILY: *Geraniaceae*
PARTS USED: *The leaves*
AROMA: *Sweet & floral; fresh & green; slightly citrus & spicy*
ENERGY: *Cool & moist*
MAIN ELEMENT: *Water (& Earth)*
PROPERTIES: *Analgesic, anti-bacterial, antidiabetic, antifungal, anti-infectious, anti-inflammatory, antispasmodic, astringent, calmative, cicatrisant, haemostatic, hepatic stimulant, insect repellent, lymphatic decongestant, pancreatic stimulant, phlebotonic, sexual tonic*
SAFETY DATA: *Non-toxic; non-irritant*

body as whole. In terms of its action on the Spleen-pancreas, the oil may be used to alleviate lethargy, diarrhoea, and lymphatic congestion. As a tonic of the *yin*, it is indicated for chronic anxiety, infertility, and symptoms associated with the menopause. It is the *cool, moist, yin-tonifying* nature of geranium that benefits dry and inflamed conditions of the skin (when applied at a dilution of only 1%).

The energetic actions of the oil can be related in turn to its psychological benefits. Clearing *heat* and smoothing the flow of *Qi*, geranium, like lavender, is able to relax the mind, calm agitation, and ease frustration and irritability. An astringent and tonic of the *yin*, it has, in addition, a consolidating, "centring" effect.

Conveying a feeling of calm strength and security, geranium oil is therefore beneficial for both chronic and acute anxiety, particularly where there is nervous exhaustion due to stress and overwork.

The oil's exotic, floral, and slightly spicy aroma is reflected in its well-known aphrodisiac effect – an effect that relates to its intrinsically sensual, liberating nature. Nourishing the feminine creativity of the Intellect *(Yi)*, and the still, receptive aspect of the the Will *(Zhi)*, geranium oil is ideal for the workaholic perfectionist – for the person who has forgotten imagination, intuition, and sensory experience.

While lavender oil is suited to the individual in whom emotions overwhelm the mind, geranium oil is for those whose rationality and personal drive deny the place of feeling and impression. The oil therefore helps to reconnect us to our feeling-life – to our emotional sensitivity, relaxed spontaneity, and healthy thirst for pleasure and enjoyment. With this comes a greater capacity for intimate communication – one in which being able to receive and experience is as important as the power to give and express.

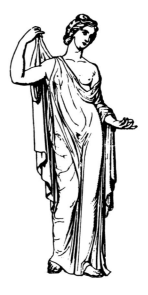

APHRODITE, GODDESS OF LOVE
As the Greek goddess of love, beauty, and fertility, Aphrodite exemplifies those aspects of the psyche that geranium oil brings to the fore. These are the more archetypically feminine qualities of sensuality, feeling, and creative intuition.

Ginger

initiative Ø self-confidence Ø accomplishment

Ginger is a tropical perennial herb, growing 60 to 120 centimetres (two to four feet) high, with reed-like stems, lanceolate leaves, and yellow flowers with purple markings. The stem grows directly from the thick tuberous rhizome, from which both the famous spice and essential oil are produced. Native to Southeast Asia, the plant grows in tropical countries throughout the world.

Ginger has been used for centuries in Asia for both culinary and medicinal purposes. In traditional Chinese medicine, the fresh root, known as *sheng jiang*, is used for colds and chills, both to promote sweating and expel mucus. The dried root, called *gan jiang*, is a major restorative of the body's *yang* energy.

Ginger was one of the first products to travel the "spice route" from Asia to Europe, where both the Greeks and Romans made extensive use of it. The Greek physician Dioscorides, in his text, *On Therapeutic Substances* (AD 77), recommended it as a digestive stimulant – a property still recognized today through the widespread use of ginger for nausea and travel sickness. In the 16th century the Spanish *conquistadores* introduced the cultivation of ginger in the West Indies, where it rapidly naturalized. Jamaican ginger is still considered the best variety for culinary use.

Therapeutically, ginger oil is essentially warming, invigorating, and decongesting. Its sphere of action is very wide – stimulating and tonifying the *yang* energy of Spleen, Stomach, Heart, Lungs, and Kidneys. It is excellent for *cold*, debilitated individuals who have a pale, swollen tongue.

Stimulating and warming the digestive organs, ginger oil is indicated for poor appetite, indigestion, abdominal distention, and flatulence. Its ability to relieve nausea makes it useful for travel and morning sickness, especially when combined with orange, Roman chamomile, and coriander oils.

As a circulatory stimulant and tonic of the Heart, ginger oil is indicated for cold hands and feet, cardiac fatigue, and angina pectoris. Its *hot*, invigorating nature makes it, in addition, a powerful rubefacient for rheumatic pain of the *cold*, contracting type.

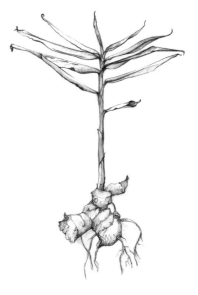

GINGER
Zingiber officinalis
FAMILY: *Zingiberaceae*
PARTS USED: *The fresh or dried rhizome*
AROMA: *Spicy, pungent, warm, sweet & woody*
ENERGY: *Hot & dry*
MAIN ELEMENT: *Water (& Fire)*
PROPERTIES: *Analgesic, anticatarrhal, aperitive, carminative, digestive stimulant, expectorant, rubefacient, sexual tonic, general tonic, stomachic*
SAFETY DATA: *Non-toxic; non-irritant*

Warming and stimulating the Lungs, ginger oil has an expectorant action suited to chronic bronchitis involving white or clear mucus. Combined with essential oils of eucalyptus, tea tree, and marjoram, it can be used to counteract colds and influenza characterized by chills, fatigue, and muscular aching. A tonic of the immune system, it will also help to prevent their recurrence.

Ginger oil's ability to strengthen the *yang-energy* of the Kidneys makes it helpful for relieving lower backache, mainly when associated with muscular fatigue. According to Oriental medicine, it is ginger's tonifying effect on the Kidneys which accounts, in addition, for its action as a sexual tonic. It may be used for impotence and frigidity in those who suffer from chronic fatigue.

The effect of ginger on the Kidneys, and more specifically the Will *(Zhi)*, also helps to account for its psychotherapeutic actions. Traditionally associated with the astrological planet Mars – a symbol of force and virility – this dynamic, fiery essence activates will-power, stimulates initiative, and restores determination. With a concomitant action on the Heart and the Mind *(Shen)*, it can in addition help to boost confidence and morale, particularly in those with poor vitality.

Ginger oil is therefore indicated for those who may have clear plans and good intentions, but who lack the personal drive and optimism to manifest initiative and take real or immediate action. Such individuals tend to procrastinate and doubt themselves, waiting for others to spur them on. They are frequently disconnected from their physical body, and may shy away from vigorous and sustained activity. Their sexual energy is often at a low ebb; a problem which may result in depression.

Ginger oil for such people is the ideal catalyst of the Will *(Zhi)*, invoking and enhancing their vital fire. Tapping this, the source of all action, ginger can restore the exhilaration of achievement.

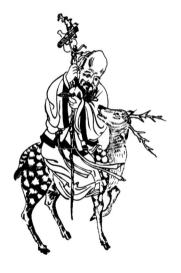

CHINESE GOD OF LONGEVITY
Ginger has for centuries been valued by the Chinese for its ability to promote strength and ensure a long life. It formed part of a medical tradition that was geared not just toward curing disease, but to assisting the art of longevity. Gentle and smiling in his yellow robe, the God of Longevity was considered the supreme disposer of earthly things.

Grapefruit

disperse ◊ lighten ◊ revive

The grapefruit is derived from a cultivated tree that, growing to a height of ten metres (32 feet), has large, glossy, dark-green leaves and white, star-shaped flowers. The origin of the tree, as well as the name, is uncertain, though it is thought to be a hybrid of the sweet orange *(Citrus sinensis)* and the pomelo, or shaddock *(Citrus maximus).*

The pomelo was brought to Spain from tropical Asia by Arab traders in the 12th century, via the same route that the orange traveled. From there it was introduced into the West Indies by the mysterious Captain Shaddock, in the 18th century. This soon lead, following its hybridization, to the New World cultivation of the grapefruit. Most of the varieties of grapefruit now grown commercially originated in Florida, where the industry first developed.

Essential oil of grapefruit is extracted through cold expression from the fresh peel of the fruit. Apart from its use in aromatherapy, it serves as a fragrance component in perfumes, cosmetics, and soaps, and as a food flavouring. Most grapefruit oil is produced in California.

Like essential oil of lemon, grapefruit is cooling, cleansing, and decongesting, and is beneficial for both an overheated Liver and a sluggish lymphatic system.

When both *heat* and stagnant *Qi-energy* have accumulated in the Liver, problems such as abdominal distention, constipation, and nausea can occur. These may be accompanied by a bitter taste in the mouth and a feeling of general irritability. Grapefruit oil will help to relieve these symptoms by regulating and cooling the Liver, and decongesting and "moving" the bowel.

A mild diuretic and stimulant of the Spleen and lymph, grapefruit oil helps the body to eliminate excess fluids and break down fats. *Dry,* sour, and decongesting, it is indicated for fluid retention, cellulite, weight gain, and obesity.

According to Oriental medicine, the individual with a *hot, damp* constitution is also prone to arteriosclerosis and hypertension (high blood pressure). Grapefruit oil, like those of lemon and melissa, is recommended to help prevent such

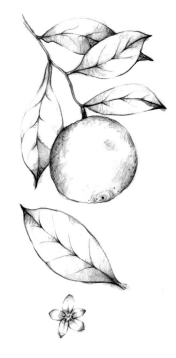

GRAPEFRUIT
Citrus paradisii
FAMILY: *Rutaceae*
PARTS USED: *The rind*
AROMA: *Fresh, light, citrus, and slightly sweet.*
ENERGY: *Cool & dry*
MAIN ELEMENT: *Wood (& Earth)*
PROPERTIES: *Aerial antiseptic, carminative, choleretic, depurative, digestive stimulant, lymphatic decongestant, stomachic*
SAFETY DATA: *Phototoxic: avoid exposure to direct sunlight or sunbed rays for 12 hours following application of the diluted essential oil to the skin*

conditions, as well as to be of benefit when they occur. Helping to purify the blood, grapefruit oil is also indicated for rheumatic pain, principally of a *hot* nature. This is when the joints feel warm and swollen, and pain is intermingled with a burning sensation.

Finally, grapefruit oil's astringent, cleansing quality makes it useful for oily skin, acne, and stretch marks.

Like other citrus oils, grapefruit's ability to smooth the flow of stagnant *Qi-energy* benefits, on a psychological level, feelings of tension, frustration, irritability, and moodiness. The oil is particularly suited to those individuals who, tense and under pressure, resort to "comfort eating" as a means of dealing with difficult emotions.

Such people have high expectations – of life, of others, and of themselves. Whenever reality fails to match up to their goals and desires, or they feel let down by others, they tend to react with anger, blame, and self-criticism. Such feelings are often followed by those of guilt and depression, and an urge to pacify and comfort the hidden vulnerable part of themselves, the criticized or shamed "inner child". Over-indulging in food and alcohol, especially sweets, chocolate, and biscuits, is the most common result of their need for comfort.

Grapefruit oil clears the psychological *heat* and congestion that result from deep-seated frustration and self-blame. Essentially cleansing, clarifying, and refreshing, it works to rid the "heavy" feelings that accompany angry disappointment, allowing us to perceive and accept more realistic goals. Like lemon, it promotes a lightness of Spirit, and eases our hunger for immediate satisfaction, our often desperate need to be "full".

TO PURIFY
The medieval alchemical symbol, "to purify" captures grapefruit oil's cleansing, decongesting properties.

Hyssop

purification ∅ protection ∅ expansion

Hyssop is a bushy perennial shrub, growing 20 to 60 centimetres (seven to 22 inches) high, with small linear leaves and whorls of purple-blue, pink or white flowers. The flowers are strongly aromatic and attract swarms of bees and butterflies. Native to southern Europe and the temperate zones of Asia, the herb now grows wild throughout Europe, Russia, and North America.

Hyssop has been used as a ritual, culinary, and medicinal herb since ancient times. Highly prized by the Hebrews, it is one of the bitter herbs mentioned in the Old Testament, employed to purify the temple. Indeed, "hyssop" derives from its ancient Hebrew name, *ezob*, meaning "holy herb". A symbol of spiritual cleansing, hyssop became associated with baptism and the forgiveness of sins.

The Romans employed hyssop to protect them against the plague, and to disinfect the houses of the sick. Valued by both Dioscorides and Galen for its powerful expectorant action, hyssop featured in all the great herbals of the Middle Ages. Commonly planted in medieval monastic gardens, the herb was distilled for its essential oil, extracted and used to flavour soups, sauces, and liqueurs such as Chartreuse.

In terms of Oriental medicine, hyssop is a strong tonic of the body's warming, dynamic *yang-energy*, especially through its action on the Lungs. Like essential oil of thyme, hyssop is very *hot* and stimulating in nature, and should therefore be used in moderation. Four or five drops is sufficient for a complete aromatherapy massage.

Strengthening the Lungs and the *Defensive-Qi*, hyssop oil benefits poor vitality, breathlessness, and immune deficiency. It helps to prevent the recurrence of colds and flu, and works to fight infection. A strong expectorant and antibacterial essential oil, it can be used with eucalyptus, tea tree, and thyme for bronchitis, pharyngitis, and sinusitis. It is mainly indicated for *cold* infections characterized by clear catarrh.

Hyssop oil also strengthens the Spleen-pancreas, and stimulates and warms the digestion. In this respect it may be used for appetite loss, slow digestion, and abdominal bloating.

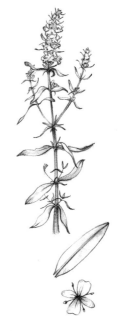

Hyssop
Hyssopus officinalis
Family: *Labiatae (Lamiaceae)*
Parts used: *The flowering tops*
Aroma: *Herbaceous, camphoraceous, warm, sweet & slightly spicy*
Energy: *Hot & dry*
Main element: *Metal*
Properties: *Antibacterial, anticatarrhal, anti-infectious, antirheumatic, antiviral, astringent, cicatrisant, decongestant, digestive stimulant, diuretic (mild), expectorant, hypertensive, immune tonic, litholytic, sudorific, general tonic, vermifuge*
Safety data: *Do not use in pregnancy or while breast-feeding, or on children under 2 yrs. Avoid using on individuals with epilepsy or fever. Do not use at more than 2% dilution*

Hyssop oil's mild diuretic action makes it useful not only for fluid retention, but to help remove the uric acid that can aggravate rheumatic conditions. Combined with oils of eucalyptus, lavender, and juniper berry, it is excellent for rheumatic pain of a *cold*, cramping nature, commonly occurring in winter.

Like most tonics of the *yang* energy, hyssop oil's effect on the nervous system and mind is a distinctly invigorating one. It is frequently recommended for poor concentration, short-term mental fatigue, and chronic nervous debility. As a tonic of the *Lung-yang* in particular, hyssop oil's rejuvenating effect on the Bodily Soul *(P'o)* also makes it helpful for melancholy and pessimism. Like thyme and eucalyptus oils, hyssop's strong, pungent aroma "opens the chest" and helps us to face the world, counteracting the urge to withdraw.

On the other hand, hyssop oil, like pine, can strengthen one's sense of personal "boundary". Traditionally considered a Herb of Protection, it was thought to defend the individual and their home from negative influences and "evil spirits". While we may consider such a view, from our modern perspective, to be a superstitious one, it is in fact the *Lung-yang* that, according to Oriental medicine, protects us both physically and psychologically. Hyssop oil therefore benefits the type of the person who is easily affected by others' moods and emotions, and who, as a result, quickly absorbs any tension in the environment.

The spiritually purifying influence of hyssop is actually quite complex. It stems from the oil's ability to sharpen awareness, "open the chest", and consolidate one's psychic field or "aura". Fully conscious and engaged, integrated and self-contained, only then are we able to feel "purged" of confused thoughts and negative emotions. Only then can we manifest the spiritual insight and generosity symbolized by Jupiter, hyssop's astrological "ruler".

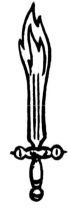

THE SWORD OF EXPULSION
While the sword generally is an ancient symbol of protection, courage, and the penetrating power of the intellect, the flaming Sword of Expulsion was an early Christian symbol of the power that guarded Paradise. Like the sword that depicted the purifying Alchemical fire, it encapsulates the purgative and empowering aspects of hyssop oil.

Jasmine

desire Ø creativity Ø harmony

Jasmine is a genus that includes some 300 species of hardy evergreen shrubs or vines, growing to a height of ten metres (32 feet). Its beautifully fragrant flowers are star-shaped and usually white or yellow in colour. Native to Northern India, Persia, and China, the plant is now widely cultivated throughout the Mediterranean and North Africa, due to its importance as a fragrance component of perfumes, soaps, and toiletries. The world's largest producer is Egypt.

Virtually all jasmine oil sold is not a true essential oil but an "absolute", produced through a process of solvent extraction rather than through steam distillation. Although the residue of the solvents employed are limited to less than ten parts per million, many still consider such concentrations sufficient to spoil the medicinal value of the oil. The alternative to jasmine absolute is oil produced through the traditional *enfleurage* process (see p.12).

Revered for centuries in the East both as a medicine and perfume, jasmine in India is called "queen of the night", because its scent is stronger after sunset. The Hindu god of love, Kama, who, like the Greek Eros and the Roman Cupid, is represented with a bow, had arrows tipped with jasmine blossoms, in order to pierce the heart with desire.

The Greek physician Dioscorides reported in the 1st century AD that the Persians used jasmine oil to perfume the air at their banquets. Along with hyacinth and rose, it also made a frequent appearance in Sufi poetry as a symbol of love and spiritual longing. The name of the plant is derived from the Persian *Yasmin*, a common name for a girl.

The therapeutic value of jasmine oil is inseparable from the exquisite, comforting sweetness of its aroma, and the effect it has on the mind and emotions. Like rose and lavender oils, it both relaxes and supports the *Qi-energy* of the Heart, calming the nerves, releasing tension, and uplifting the Mind *(Shen)*. As a result, jasmine is one of the most effective essential oils for nervous anxiety, restlessness, and depression – whether the individual involved has a *hot* or *cold, excess* or *deficient* constitution.

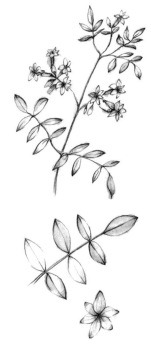

JASMINE
Jasminum officinalis
FAMILY: *Oleaceae*
PARTS USED: *The flower*
AROMA: *Warm, rich, floral & sweet*
ENERGY: *Neutral temperature/ neutral moisture*
MAIN ELEMENT: *Fire (& Water)*
PROPERTIES: *Antidepressive, calmative, emollient, lactogenic, parturient, sexual tonic, uterine tonic*
SAFETY DATA: *Non-toxic; non-irritant*

Its other main area of therapeutic influence is upon the urogenital organs, where a warming, restorative action combines with a gently decongesting one. A renowned aphrodisiac and sexual tonic, jasmine oil is indicated for impotence and frigidity, especially when there are depressive thoughts of inadequacy and undesirability. A mildly astringent decongestant, it may also be used for leucorrhoea and genital discharges generally.

Jasmine oil's reputed benefits during labour, for difficult, painful deliveries, have been shown to be relatively mild, and less effective than lavender and clary sage. However, on a psychological level, the oil is undoubtedly of value, easing the trauma of a prolonged labour, and enhancing the joy of giving birth. It may also be employed as a lactogenic, promoting the production of breast milk.

Jasmine, in traditional terms, was classified as a Fertility Herb, most obviously due to its potential as an aphrodisiac. Harmonizing the sensual aspect of our being with the emotional, jasmine is, however, much more than simply a sexual stimulant. Whenever fear and vulnerability, or anxiety and depression, cut us off from our ability to share physical pleasure and affection, jasmine oil can support, reassure, and delight. Its voluptuously warm, joyous fragrance allows the heart to flow again through the river of the senses.

If jasmine can reawaken passion and reunite it with love, so too, on a mental-spiritual level, can it restore a capacity for creativity, for "fertility of mind". With the instinctual, reflective Moon as its astrological symbol, the oil may be used to enhance intuition and the potential for original thought.

Bearing in mind its euphoric, sensual qualities, jasmine is most applicable for the kind of depression that results from unconscious restraint and repression – an approach to life based on values discordant with the individual soul and its true desires.

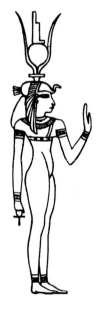

ISIS, GODDESS OF FERTILITY
Associated throughout history with the generally compassionate goddesses of the Moon, jasmine – grown along the Nile – may be represented by Isis, the Egyptian mother goddess who held the secrets of fertility, magic, and healing. She is thought to have founded the custom of marriage.

Juniper
fortify ∅ unburden ∅ empower

Among the 60 or so species that make up the genus of *Juniperus*, it is the berries of the common juniper *(Juniperus communis)* that are used as a medicine, spice, and source of essential oil. Common juniper is a prickly evergreen shrub or small tree, reaching a height of twelve metres (39 feet), with blue-green needle-like leaves, greenish-yellow flowers and small round berries. The berries change over three years from green to blue and then black. Native to northern Europe, south-west Asia and North America, juniper grows on heaths, moorland, mountain slopes, and in coniferous forests.

Juniper is one of the very first plants to be used by humankind. In fact, remains of the berries have been found at prehistoric dwelling sites in the Swiss lakes. The aromatic, antiseptic quality of the plant meant that it was commonly burnt as a fumigant and ritual incense – by the Ancient Greeks to combat epidemics, and by the Tibetans and native Americans for ceremonial purposes. Considered a panacea throughout the Middle Ages, the abbess and physician St Hildegarde von Bingen recommended a hot bath of the crushed berries for infections of the respiratory tract. During the 19th century, the berries were burnt in French hospitals to prevent the spread of smallpox.

The English name "juniper" is derived from the Latin *juniores*, meaning "young berries", while the French name for the plant, *genièvre*, is likely to originate from the Celtic words *gen*, meaning "small bush", and *prus*, meaning "hot and bitter". From *gen* came the word *gin*, one of the spirits that the juniper berry flavours.

Like essential oils of thyme and ginger, juniper is a powerful tonic of the body's warming and stimulating *yang* energy, especially of the *Kidney-yang*. It is both a diuretic and lymphatic decongestant. In respect of its action on the *Kidney-yang* and urinary system, juniper oil's warming, invigorating effect benefits chronic tiredness, cold hands and feet, lower backache, and oedema (fluid retention).

Juniper oil's diuretic property is coupled with a strengthening effect on Spleen-pancreas to make it one of the most

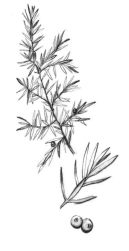

Juniper
Juniperus communis
Family: *Cupressaceae*
Parts used: *The ripe fruit*
Aroma: *Fresh, piney, balsamic, bittersweet & woody*
Energy: *Hot & dry*
Main element: *Water (& Metal)*
Properties: *Anticatarrhal, anti-infectious, antirheumatic, antiseborrhoeic, decongestant, depurative, diuretic, expectorant, lymphatic decongestant, neurotonic, rubefacient, general tonic*
Safety data: *Non-toxic; non-irritant*

powerful of aromatic decongestants. Ridding the body of *cold dampness*, it is indicated for abdominal distention, obesity, and arteriosclerosis. This type of congestion can also lead to oily skin, for which juniper oil may be applied in a base cream together with lavender and cedarwood oils.

Like hyssop, juniper berry oil's diuretic and rubefacient properties mean that it is also effective for rheumatic pain, mainly of a *cold*, cramping nature. And the oil's anti-infectious potential may be utilized against cystitis, urinary tract infection, and bronchitis, especially in those who are *cold* and congested, or wheezy and lethargic.

Juniper's piney, pungent aroma clearly associate it both energetically and psychologically with an ability to disperse and cleanse. It is no small wonder that since ancient times it has been associated with spiritual purification, as well as the power to drive out negative influences. On the other hand, the warm, sweet and woody notes of the essence reflect its deeply fortifying potential. This we can link clearly to its action on the Kidneys, and to its reinforcing effect on the Will *(Zhi)*.

Juniper works, therefore, to break through psychological stagnation and consolidate will-power. It is suited to the individual who, feeling burdened and aloof, is deeply absorbed in their own thoughts – thoughts which revolve around worries, pressures, and unpleasant memories.

Feeling unsupported and misunderstood by others, such people tend to withdraw, and lose their social confidence. The gloomy, disinterested outlook that develops can gradually become deeply embedded, producing a contraction and rigidity of Spirit that may become somatized (manifested in the body) as stiff and painful joints.

Juniper oil helps to purge us of the worry and self-absorption that is rooted in a fear of failure. Restoring our determination to overcome life's obstacles, it replaces stasis and isolation with movement and openness. It is well-represented by the astrological Mars, symbol of instinctive confidence and fire.

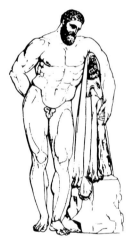

HERACLES, GREEK GOD OF STRENGTH
Like Mars and Aries, the gods of war, Heracles was a sun hero who typified strength and valour. His twelve labours, or tasks, are a mythic demonstration of the same imperturbable resolve that juniper berry oil encourages.

Laurel

inspiration ∅ self-esteem ∅ insight

Laurel, also known as "bay" or "sweet laurel", is an upright, evergreen shrub or small tree, reaching a height of twenty metres (65 feet), with dark-green lanceolate leaves and small clusters of yellow flowers. The flowers are succeeded by small, purple-black aromatic berries. Native to the Mediterranean but grown the world over, laurel is cultivated in gardens as a container-grown ornamental.

The plant's botanical name reveals the lofty stature bestowed upon it by the ancients: *laurus* from the Latin meaning "to praise", and *nobilis* meaning "renowned" or "famous". A symbol of triumph and achievement to both the Greeks and Romans, crowns of its leaves were worn by victorious generals, emperors, and poets. In medieval times scholars and graduates were crowned with wreaths of laurel, or *bacca laurea* – from which derived the French bacca-laureate (awarded on completion of one's secondary education). In the English language, the symbolism of the plant is reflected in the British Poet Laureate, as well as the phrase "to win one's laurels".

Laurel was dedicated, like rosemary, to Apollo, Greek god of light, poetry, and prophecy. It was Apollo who, according to the ancient myth, decreed that the laurel garland should be a sign of success in the arts. He did this after the mountain nymph Daphne had herself changed into a laurel tree, in order to escape the god's amorous pursuits.

At Delphi, the site of Apollo's oracle, laurel was one of the Visionary Herbs burnt by the temple priestess as part of her prophetic ritual. Believing it conferred the power of divination, the Ancient Greeks would place the leaves under a pillow to stimulate dreams of prophecy. They also considered it a Herb of Protection – against lightning, evil, and disease. This association continued well into the Middle Ages, when it became traditional practice to plant a laurel tree by the front door of the house.

The medicinal values of laurel have been recognized since ancient times. The renowned Greek physician Galen, in AD165, recommended it as a diuretic and liver stimulant,

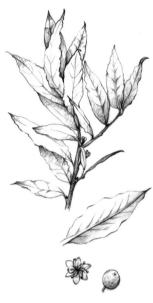

LAUREL

Laurus nobilis

FAMILY: *Lauraceae*

PARTS USED: *The leaves and branches*

AROMA: *Fresh, medicinal, camphoraceous, sweet & slightly cinnamon-like*

ENERGY: *Warm & dry*

MAIN ELEMENT: *Fire*

PROPERTIES: *Analgesic, antibacterial, anticatarrhal, antifungal, anti-infectious, antispasmodic, antirheumatic, antiviral, carminative, digestive stimulant, expectorant, neurotonic*

SAFETY DATA: *Do not use on children under 2 yrs. Avoid using on hypersensitive, diseased, or damaged skin. Do not use at more than 2% dilution*

classifying the berries and leaves of the tree as *hot* and *dry*. An infusion of the pitted, crushed berries became a traditional remedy for rheumatism and oedema (fluid retention).

Essential oil of laurel is produced from the leaves and branches, and is characterized therapeutically by antispasmodic, carminative, and expectorant properties. Energetically, its principal actions are to circulate and regulate the *Qi-energy* and to clear *cold phlegm*.

In terms of its action on the digestive system, laurel may be used together with orange, marjoram, and coriander oils for abdominal bloating, slow digestion, colic, and flatulence. As a pulmonary antiseptic and expectorant, laurel oil will relieve catarrhal colds and chronic bronchitis – combined, for example, with eucalyptus and pine. Laurel oil's diuretic and *Qi-moving* properties also make it helpful in cases of osteoarthritis and rheumatism, mainly of a *cold*, cramping nature.

Laurel's effect on a psychotherapeutic level rests both on its neurotonic action and ability to uplift the Mind *(Shen)*. Like rosemary, laurel oil may be used for poor concentration, lack of memory, and chronic nervous debility. It is particularly indicated for chilly, congested individuals who lack energy and confidence.

While rosemary helps to restore purpose and direction by strengthening self-identity, laurel oil works in a similar way, through stimulating inspiration and creative boldness. It is suited to individuals who, lacking in self-esteem, doubt their abilities, intellectual and otherwise. It is this very doubt – this self-imposed limitation – that can inhibit their capacity for intuitive thought.

Laurel oil assists by stimulating both the rational and "higher mind", and by helping to renew one's belief in one's own boundless potential. This it does principally through re-igniting the Fire Element, where its fresh and spicy scent elevates the Spirit and sparks our inner vision.

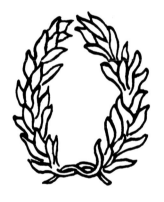

THE LAUREL WREATH
The laurel tree was a Graeco-Roman symbol of both triumph and peace, and, because it was evergreen, represented immortality. It was sacred to Apollo, whose high moral and intellectual status ensured his place as the principal cultivator of civilization.

$\mathcal{L}$avender

calm composure Ø easy self-expression

Lavender is a hardy fragrant shrub, growing to a height of one metre (three feet), with narrow, lanceolate leaves and grey-blue flowers in terminal spikes, borne on slender stalks. While the fine aroma of lavender is found throughout the plant, the essential oil can be extracted only from its flowers.

Indigenous to the mountainous areas of Mediterranean Europe, the plant is now cultivated the world over, growing best on poor, well-drained soils. The major producers of the essential oil are Bulgaria, France, Croatia, and Russia.

Among the numerous varieties of lavender grown, the most important are spike lavender *(Lavandula spica),* French lavender *(Lavandula stoechas)* and true, or English, lavender *(Lavandula officinalis,* also known as *Lav. angustifolia* and *Lav. vera).* True lavender is the most important medicinally, while spike lavender was the plant used by the Ancient Romans to scent their bath water. In fact, the name "lavender" is derived from the Latin *lavare,* meaning "to wash".

Lavender is the best known "nose herb", prized for its fresh, soft fragrance since antiquity. Recommended by Dioscorides for "ye griefs in ye thorax", it later earned considerable attention from St Hildegarde von Bingen, who recommended it for "maintaining a pure character". In 1660, Richard Surflet wrote that the "distilled water of the flowers restoreth the lost speech, and healeth the swoonings and disease of the heart".

In terms of Oriental medicine, the *cool,* dispersing, and relaxing qualities of lavender benefit *heat* and inflammation, spasm and pain, and general unrest. The antiseptic qualities of the oil also make it suitable for a wide range of infections.

Like German chamomile, lavender oil works to regulate and cool an overheated Liver, relieving headache, migraine, constipation, and general irritability. Soothing and supporting the *Qi-energy* of the Heart, the oil may also be used in the treatment of nervous tension, insomnia, palpitations, and high blood pressure.

The antispasmodic, analgesic nature of the essential oil benefits problems as diverse as colic and irritable bowel, premenstrual tension and menstrual pain, and muscular stiffness

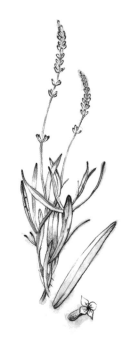

LAVENDER
Lavandula officinalis
(syn. angustifolia/ vera)
FAMILY: *Labiatae (Lamiaceae)*
PART USED: *The flower*
AROMA: *Fresh & herbaceous; soft & floral; bittersweet*
ENERGY: *Cool & dry*
MAIN ELEMENT: *Fire (& Wood)*
PROPERTIES: *Analgesic, antibacterial, antifungal, anti-infectious, anti-inflammatory, antirheumatic, antispasmodic, calmative, cardiotonic, cholagogic, cicatrisant, hypotensive, vermifuge*
SAFETY DATA: *Non-toxic; non-irritant*

and aching. In addition, its gentle anti-infectious qualities make it useful for genito-urinary and respiratory infections.

Applied with wet cotton wool, lavender oil may soothe mild burns, and added to a cream, gel, or milk base, used in the treatment of inflammatory skin conditions such as dermatitis, psoriasis, and eczema.

The psychological uses of lavender oil stem from its ability to calm and stabilize the *Qi* of the Heart. The home of the Mind *(Shen)*, the Heart is responsible for maintaining our overall mental-emotional equilibrium. Supporting the Heart in this central function, the oil can ease nervous tension and allay feelings of panic and hysteria. As John Gerard wrote in 1597, lavender "doth help the passion and panting of the heart". An aromatic "Rescue Remedy", it works to calm any strong emotions that threaten to overwhelm the mind.

Lavender oil helps, in addition, to release pent-up energy within the Wood Element, smoothing the flow of *Qi-energy* and so easing frustration and irritability. By releasing mental energy that has become "stuck" in habitual behaviour – especially when it results from a build-up of unexpressed emotion – lavender has been described by herbalist Peter Holmes as "both habit-breaker and crisis smoother".

The feeling of calmness and composure that the oil instils is evoked by the closed-in, almost self-protective, appearance of lavender's radiant blue flowers. It is the kind of self-possessed equanimity symbolized by the plant's astrological "ruler", the sign of Virgo. And just as the characteristics of Virgo include over-sensitivity and inhibition, so too can lavender calm the nervous anxiety that results in shyness and embarrassment.

Soothing the sense of trauma that inhibits self-expression, lavender is suited to the individual who is full of creative potential, but who is frustrated in fulfilling it due to self-conscious reserve. It therefore encourages the full expression and perfection of the individual self that the sixth sign of the Zodiac symbolizes.

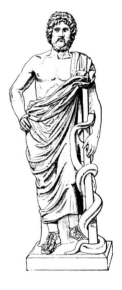

AESCLEPIUS, GOD OF MEDICINE
The wide and renowned healing powers of lavender oil are best represented by the Greek god of healing, Aesclepius. The son of Apollo, Aesclepius was raised by Chiron, the centaur whose knowledge encompassed the arts and sciences, including the secrets of medicine.

Lemon

refreshing ◊ clear ◊ trusting

Citrus limonum is a small evergreen tree, growing three to six metres high (nine to 19 feet), with pale-green ovate leaves and highly perfumed white and pink flowers. An individual tree can produce as many as 1,500 lemons per year, each fruit turning from green to yellow as it ripens.

Like the other citrus trees, the lemon tree originated in Asia. Finding its way to Greece in the 2nd century AD, it made little impact in Europe until the Middle Ages, when it was cultivated in Spain and Sicily. It grows today throughout the Mediterranean, though Florida and California are the largest producers of the oil.

Referred to by the Roman historian Virgil as the "median apple", the peel was used in ancient times to perfume clothes and repel insects. However, it was not until the late 17th century that the neo-Galenic pharmacist Nicholas Lemery gave full recognition to the medicinal value of the fruit. In his book of 1698, he mentions lemon as being both an effective blood cleanser and carminative. When the British Navy issued large quantities of the fruit to counteract the onslaught of scurvy on lengthy sea voyages, its reputation grew. In Spain and other European countries, lemon became widely known as a panacea, especially where toxicity and infection were involved.

Produced through the cold expression of the outer peel of the fruit, the essential oil is one of the lightest in aromatherapy, an example of a predominantly "top note" fragrance. Like bergamot and grapefruit oils, the only caution as to its normal use is its potential phototoxicity.

In terms of Oriental medicine, lemon oil is *cool* and *dry* in nature, and clears *heat, dampness,* and *phlegm.* It is one of the best essential oils to decongest, cleanse, and detoxify.

Like grapefruit oil, lemon's ability to clear *hot dampness* and *phlegm* is reflected in its action as a lymphatic decongestant. It is indicated in this respect for obesity, cellulite, high blood cholesterol, and arteriosclerosis. It is also considered to have a litholytic potential to help remove urinary stones and gallstones. Clearing *heat* and toxicity from a congested,

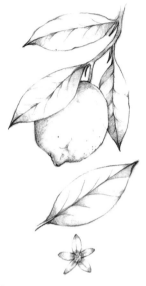

LEMON
Citrus limonum
FAMILY: *Rutaceae*
PARTS USED: *The rind*
AROMA: *Fresh, light, citrus, sour, and slightly sweet*
ENERGY: *Cool & dry*
MAIN ELEMENT: *Earth (& Fire)*
PROPERTIES: *Antibacterial, anti-coagulant, anti-infectious, anti-inflammatory, antifungal, antirheumatic, antisclerotic, antispasmodic, antiviral, astringent, calmative, carminative, digestive stimulant, diuretic (mild), hypotensive, immune tonic, litholytic, lymphatic decongestant, pancreatic stimulant, phlebotonic, stomachic*
SAFETY DATA: *Phototoxic: avoid exposure to direct sunlight or sunbed rays for 12 hours following application of the diluted essential oil to the skin*

overworked Liver, the oil in addition can help to relieve nausea, headaches, irritability, and insomnia.

The anticoagulant property of lemon oil is described in energetic terms as an ability to *move the blood* – a therapeutic effect that depends partly on its astringent nature. Improving circulation and toning the blood vessels, the oil may be used for broken capillaries, varicose veins, haemorrhoids, and nosebleeds. It is also appropriate for people with hypertension, especially when combined with lavender, neroli, and melissa oils.

Lemon oil's antiviral nature makes it helpful for colds and flu, especially when characterized by yellow or green catarrh. Its generally anti-infectious property also make it an excellent aerial antiseptic – one that can be sprayed in hospital wards, creches, and around the home.

Lemon oil's effectiveness for conditions of *dampness* and *phlegm* depend partly on its action on the Spleen-pancreas. It is the energetic role of the Spleen to transform food and drink, and when it fails to do so efficiently such congestion is often the result. A pancreatic stimulant and mental decongestant, lemon oil acts mainly on the Earth Element.

With its bright, sour scent, lemon oil sharpens the focus of consciousness, clarifying and uplifting the Intellect *(Yi)*. It calms, lightens, and refreshes, dispersing confusion and easing worry. Reducing mental plethora, it rescues a mind bogged down by burdens, decisions, and obstacles.

Lemon is associated with the planets of both human and divine love – Venus and Neptune – and has long been considered a mild aphrodisiac. Its ability to uplift and clarify affects not only the Intellect *(Yi)* but the Heart and Mind *(Shen)* as well. Dispersing and "cooling" emotional confusion and doubt, lemon oil can encourage greater trust and security. Like oil of rose, it can help to "open the heart" – by alleviating fears of emotional involvement and of losing oneself in another person.

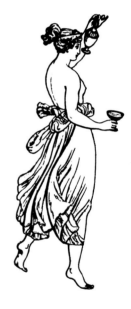

HEBE, GODDESS OF YOUTH
The long reputation of lemon as a panacea and preserver of good health makes Hebe, the Greek goddess of youth, a suitably fresh-faced emblem for both the fruit and its oil. The gods' cup-bearer, she became the wife of Heracles after he completed his twelve labours.

Marjoram

comfort Ø contentment Ø compassion

Sweet marjoram is an aromatic herb, growing 30-80 centi-metres (11 to 31 inches) high, with dark-green ovate leaves and spiky clusters of small flowers, white to pink in colour. The entire flowering herb is distilled for its essential oil. Native to southern Europe and the Near East, the plant is cultivated throughout Europe and North Africa, the largest producers of the oil being France and Egypt. Pot marjoram *(Origanum onites)* is a variety that is cultivated in areas too cold for *Origanum marjorana*, while wild marjoram *(Origanum vulgare)* is the true oregano of the herb garden.

The generic name *Origanum* is derived from the Greek words *oros* and *ganos*, meaning "joy of the mountains". The Old French name for the plant, *mariol*, alludes to the knots of flowers that are thought to resemble little marionettes.

Sweet, wild, and pot marjoram have been widely used since ancient times, for both culinary and medicinal purposes. Cultivated by the Ancient Egyptians, pot marjoram was used to make perfumes, unguents, and medicines, and was dedi-cated to Osiris, the dying-and-rising god who was king of the afterlife and overlord of agriculture.

To the Greeks, wild marjoram was a Funeral Herb, planted on graves to bring spiritual peace to the departed. Associated with Aphrodite, goddess of love, beauty, and fertility, it was also a symbol of love and honour, and the flowers were used to crown young married couples. It was said that the plant was given scent by Aphrodite's gentle touch.

The 1st-century Greek physician Dioscorides, a widely experienced army doctor, himself made an ointment of mar-joram called *amaricimum*, to warm and strengthen the nerves. Recognition of the plant's restorative powers contin-ued throughout history; in Tudor times in England even the smell of it was believed to keep one healthy.

Sweet marjoram is one of the main essential oils that pos-sess an ability to both strengthen and relax. In terms of Oriental medicine, marjoram tonifies and circulates *Qi-energy*, clears *cold phlegm*, and calms the mind. Marjoram oil's *Qi-moving* action results in its very distinct antispasmod-

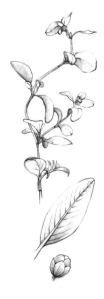

SWEET MARJORAM
Origanum marjorana
FAMILY: *Labiatae (Lamiaceae)*
PARTS USED: *The whole flowering herb*
AROMA: *Fresh & herbaceous; warm & camphoraceous; sweet & slightly woody*
ENERGY: *Warm & dry*
MAIN ELEMENT: *Earth (& Fire)*
PROPERTIES: *Analgesic, anti-bacterial, anti-infectious, antispas-modic, calmative, carminative, digestive stimulant, diuretic (mild), expectorant, hypotensive, neurotonic, stomachic, vasodilator*
SAFETY DATA: *Non-toxic; non-irritant*

ic and analgesic properties. It may be applied in this respect for conditions such as muscular stiffness and pain, nervous spasm, intestinal colic, and osteoarthritis. Smoothing the flow of *Qi-energy* in the chest, it can also be used to calm and regulate the heart, making it indicated for palpitations, tachycardia, and hypertension. Its antispasmodic action on the chest means, in addition, that it is one of the best essential oils for a nervous cough and asthma, particularly when there is white or clear catarrh.

In terms of its tonifying, strengthening influence, marjoram may be used for both chronic lethargy and nervous exhaustion. It is especially helpful for conditions in which tiredness alternates with tension, or is characterized by anxiety or insomnia. Restoring the *Qi* of the Spleen-pancreas, yet calming the nerves, marjoram is innately "balancing".

It is the sweet, nourishing, and balancing quality of marjoram, together with its regulating effect on the Intellect *(Yi)*, that associate marjoram primarily with the Earth Element. Whenever the Earth Element is depleted or under stress, worry and overthinking can take hold. There may, in addition, be feelings of real or imagined emotional deprivation – the idea that "no one cares". Regardless of whether the person is truly isolated or not, they tend to see themselves as lonely and unsupported, easily feeling denied both warmth and affection.

Relaxing, warming, and comforting, marjoram oil addresses itself to each aspect of this psychological picture. It helps to calm obsessive thinking, ease emotional craving and promote the capacity for inner self-nurturing. In its ancient role as a Funeral Herb, it can help us to accept any deep loss, especially when combined with oils of cypress and rose. As a Herb of Love, it nourishes the place from where neediness springs, helping to restore our power to give. A distillation of Mother Earth's compassion, marjoram oil shows us "the joy of the mountains".

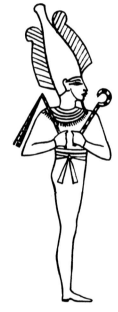

OSIRIS, KING OF ETERNITY
The Ancient Egyptians utilized marjoram – a traditional Funeral Herb – in the worship of Osiris. As lord of the afterlife, it was Osiris who sat in judgment over those who entered his domain, by weighing their hearts against the feather of truth.

Melissa

gentle strength Ø fearless serenity

Also known as "balm" or "lemon balm", melissa is a lemony sweet-scented perennial herb, growing 30 to 60 centimetres (11 to 23 inches) high, with bright-green, oval- to heart-shaped leaves and small, loose clusters of white, pink, or yellowish flowers. Native to the Mediterranean, melissa is now cultivated in gardens the world over. Revered since ancient times, its name derives from the Greek *melittena*, or "honey-bee", because, according to Dioscorides, "the bees do delight in the herb". Cultivated as a bee plant, its abundant nectar helps to produce some of the very best honey.

Both Dioscorides and the Roman medical botanist Pliny noted melissa's analgesic, antispasmodic, and vulnerary properties, recommending it for toothache, asthma, and wounds. Highly valued by Arabian physicians, Avicenna, in his 11th-century materia medica, *The Canon of Medicine*, "teacheth that balm maketh the heart merry and joyful, and strengtheneth the vital spirits". This reflects the ancient reputation it held for easing cardiac and nervous disorders, and, above all, for counteracting melancholy. Widely considered to promote longevity, the Swiss-born physician and alchemist Paracelsus (1493-1541) called it "The Elixir of Life".

A great deal of "melissa oil" currently being sold is not essential oil of true *Melissa officinalis* at all. It is often a blend of lemongrass and citronella, together with naturally derived chemicals similar to the constituents of the real product. These false, reconstructed versions of the oil appear because the real thing is so expensive – due to the very small amount of essence that can be extracted from fresh melissa leaves. One should check, therefore, with suppliers or retailers, that the oil is produced from *Melissa officinalis* alone. If it is, it won't be cheap! The gentle power of this unique essential oil nevertheless makes it well worth the investment.

Energetically *cool* and *dry*, melissa oil is indicated for stagnation of *Qi-energy*, for *heat* in the Liver and Heart, and for disturbance of the Mind *(Shen)*.

Melissa's ability to circulate stagnant *Qi-energy* is reflected in its well-known antispasmodic, digestive properties.

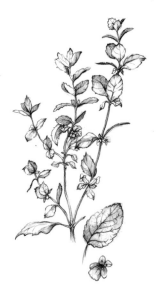

MELISSA

Melissa officinalis

FAMILY: *Labiatae (Lamiaceae)*

PARTS USED: *The leaves*

AROMA: *Fresh, green, herbaceous, citrus & slightly sweet*

ENERGY: *Cool & dry*

MAIN ELEMENT: *Fire (& Wood)*

PROPERTIES: *Analgesic, anti depressive, anti-inflammatory, antispasmodic, calmative, carminative, choleretic, digestive stimulant, hypotensive, litholytic, vasodilator*

SAFETY DATA: *Do not use in pregnancy or while breast-feeding, or on children under 2 yrs. Avoid using on hypersensitive, diseased, or damaged skin and on those with prostatic hyperplasia or glaucoma. Do not use at more than 1% dilution*

Enhancing the function of the Liver, Stomach, and intestines, the oil may be used for epigastric spasm, nervous indigestion, nausea, and flatulence. Smoothing the flow of *Qi-energy* in the Lungs, it is also indicated for conditions of nervous asthma, and alleviates coughs and bronchitis with yellowish catarrh. Like lavender oil, its analgesic property means that it can relieve migraine and menstrual pain.

Melissa oil's cooling, soothing action on the Heart and nerves benefits restlessness, insomnia, and nervous agitation. A vasodilator, it is also recommended for hypertension.

Harmonizing both the Mind *(Shen)* and the Ethereal Soul *(Hun)*, melissa oil is important for depression – particularly in those who are emotionally sensitive and do not respond well to pressure. Itself a plant of a gentle yet hardy disposition, its subtle effect resonates with people who are easily traumatized by confrontation. They tend to manifest their strength through trying to contain, rather than respond to and express, feelings of hurt and anger. These emotions therefore build up within, generating an oppressive state of mind described by Nicholas Culpeper, the 17th century herbalist, as "black choler".

According to Culpeper, melissa is represented by the fourth sign of the Zodiac, Cancer. Apart from "ruling" the pericardium, breasts, and stomach, Cancer is symbolic of our emotional roots – of mothering and childhood. Melissa can reach the deepest layers of the psyche, the "inner child" of our emotional being. With its lemon-fresh honey-like sweetness, it can help to restore both clarity and security to a confused, dependent soul.

Just as lavender calms the emotions when they overwhelm the mind, melissa oil, in a similar way, replaces intensity with serenity, and distrust with innocence. As its sour, astringent quality "reabsorbs" the Mind *(Shen)* into the Heart – its stable residence and foundation – melissa is the most effective oil for anxious depression and a feeling of foreboding.

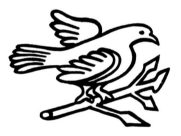

THE DOVE OF PEACE
The dove is an ancient symbol of peace, gentleness, and purity, as well as of femininity and maternity. The Christian image here reminds us of melissa oil's ability to restore tranquillity and simplicity of heart, and yet provide a source of spiritual strength.

Myrrh

tranquil solitude Ø transcendent peace

Myrrh is the resinous exudation, or gum, collected from one of 80 or so species of the *Commiphora* genus, the thorny, stunted shrubs that grow in the Middle East, northern India, and North Africa. Reaching a height of three metres (nine feet), *Commiphora molmol* has numerous knotted branches, scanty trifoliate leaves, and small white flowers. Through fissures in its bark, the trunk exudes a pale-yellow oleoresin, hardening to semi-transparent, reddish-brown "tears" on exposure to air.

A derivation of the Arabic *murr*, meaning "bitter", the gum has been used throughout the Near East and Mediterranean for almost four millennia. It was one of the very first aromatic substances valued for its rich and enduring scent.

Myrrh played a central role in the religious and medical life of the Ancient Egyptians, who called it "punt" or "phun". They used it both as an ingredient of healing unguents as well as a revered Funeral Herb, burning it as an incense to honour the dead. It was said to come from the tears of Horus, the falcon-headed sun god.

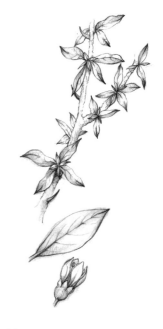

MYRRH
Commiphora molmol
FAMILY: *Burseraceae*
PARTS USED: *The gum*
AROMA: *Resinous, balsamic, rich & slightly camphoraceous*
ENERGY: *Warm & dry*
MAIN ELEMENT: *Earth (& Metal)*
PROPERTIES: *Antibacterial, anti-catarrhal, antidepressive, anti-infectious, anti-inflammatory, antiparasitic, antiviral, astringent, balsamic, calmative, carminative, cicatrisant, expectorant, vulnerary*
SAFETY DATA: *Non-toxic; non-irritant*

Myrrh was of equal importance to the Ancient Hebrews, who drank it with wine to prepare themselves for religious ceremonies, in order to raise their consciousness. Not only was myrrh present at the birth of Christ – as one of the Magi's three gifts – but at his death as well. In *The Gospel According to St John*, Nicodemus, before the burial of Jesus, "brought a mixture of myrrh and aloes, then took the body of Jesus, and wound it in linen clothes with the spices, as the manner of the Jews is to bury".

Valued therapeutically throughout history, myrrh found its way into ointments and salves of all kinds, from Greek and Roman times to the 20th century. It was consistently used for its antiseptic, vulnerary, and anticatarrhal properties.

In terms of Oriental medicine, myrrh is *warm* and *dry* in energy. The oil benefits those who are lethargic, cold, and congested due a weakness of the Spleen-pancreas and a resulting accumulation of *dampness*. Astringent in nature, it is therefore indicated for chronic diarrhoea and vaginal discharges. Clinical research has shown that the gum also helps to lower blood cholesterol levels, benefiting those with obesity and ischaemic heart disease.

Myrrh oil is also known for its antibacterial, antifungal, and anti-inflammatory actions, and has been traditionally employed in the treatment of mouth, gum, and throat infections, as well as vaginitis and thrush. Its balsamic-expectorant property makes it indicated for laryngitis, loss of voice, and bronchitis, particularly when combined with eucalyptus, tea tree, and pine essential oils.

Like frankincense oil, myrrh's effect on the nervous system is a gently calming one, able to instil deep tranquillity of mind. With its sweet, resinous, and earthy base-note aroma, together with its effect on the Spleen-pancreas, myrrh can be associated mainly with the Element Earth. Soothing, clarifying, and grounding the Intellect *(Yi)*, it is one the principal oils for overthinking, worry, and mental distraction.

Myrrh oil's effect on the Spirit – again, like frankincense – is one of inner stillness and peace, of an awareness freed from the restless and mundane. As a Funeral Herb, the peace that the oil conveys gives it the ability to ease sorrow and grief – linking it, in addition, to the Metal Element. Vulnerary in nature – appearing when the plant is wounded – myrrh subtly helps to close the wounds of both loss and rejection. A distillation of the desert's eternal landscape, the oil embodies the soothing power of solitude.

As an ancient esoteric Magical Herb, myrrh unites the spiritual with the physical. Building a bridge between "Heaven" and "Earth", it strengthens the link between our crown and base chakras – the psychic centres at the base of the spine and top of the head. By so doing, the dreams and visions of the soul can find a channel for earthly expression, and tap the force they need for their "magical" realization.

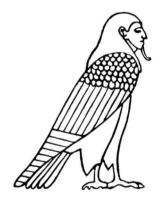

BA, THE SELF
The effect of myrrh oil reaches far into the psyche, and can help us to both transcend and transform aspects of material existence. It heightens our awareness of the Self, which, to the Ancient Egyptians, was depicted as the bird-like Ba-soul, formless and free. It was distinguished from the Ka-soul of the intellect and ego.

Neroli

reassurance ◊ retrieval ◊ renewal

Neroli is extracted from the fragrant flowers of the bitter orange tree, also known as the sour or Seville orange tree (*Citrus aurantium var. amara*, or *Citrus bigaradia*). The evergreen tree, growing to a height of ten metres (32 feet), has dark-green, ovate leaves, white flowers with thick, fleshy petals, and small, dark fruits.

Native to Southeast Asia – from where it spread to India and Persia – the tree today grows in the Mediterranean, California, and South America. It is one of the few plants that produce more than one essential oil: neroli from the blossoms, petitgrain from the leaves and twigs, and bitter orange oil from the rind of the fruit. The major producers of neroli oil are Tunisia, Italy, and France.

The bitter orange was first cultivated in the Mediterranean by Arab conquerors in the 10th or 11th century. After the discovery of the New World, the tree was introduced to the West Indies, and then to North, Central, and South America. However, it was not until 1563 that the distilled oil of the blossoms is mentioned, recorded by the Italian naturalist della Porta.

Neroli is thought to have been named after Anna Maria de la Tremoille, Princess of Neroli (near Rome), who in the 17th century introduced the oil to Italian society. Anna Maria used the scent wherever she could – on her gloves, stationery, and scarves.

Neroli was also employed as a scent by the prostitutes of Madrid, so they would be recognized by its aroma. On the other hand, the blossoms were worn as a bridal headdress and carried as a bouquet, symbolizing purity and virginity. Together with lavender, bergamot, lemon, and rosemary oils, neroli was a key constituent of the classic toilet water eau-de-Cologne. Medicinally, it was valued as a gentle tonic of the nervous system.

Cool in temperature and neutral in moisture, neroli oil clears *heat*, relaxes the nerves, and uplifts the Spirit.

Together with rose, lavender, and melissa, it is one of the best essential oils to calm and stabilize the Heart and Mind

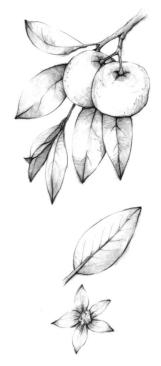

NEROLI
Citrus aurantium var. amara
FAMILY: *Rutaceae*
PARTS USED: *The flower*
AROMA: *Floral, bittersweet, warm, rich & orange-like*
ENERGY: *Cool temperature/ neutral moisture*
MAIN ELEMENT: *Fire (& Wood)*
PROPERTIES: *Antibacterial, antidepressive, anti-infectious, antiparasitic, astringent (mild), calmative, digestive stimulant, phlebotonic*
SAFETY DATA: *Non-toxic; non-irritant*

(Shen). Neroli is particularly good for *hot*, agitated conditions of the Heart characterized by restlessness, insomnia, and palpitations, and is indicated for hypertension (high blood pressure). An all-round regulator of the nervous system, neroli oil helps to ease mental and emotional tension, nervous depression, and both chronic and acute anxiety.

With an action similar to that of orange peel oil, neroli is also of benefit to the Liver and Spleen-pancreas, and regulates nervous dyspepsia, abdominal spasm, and colic. Mildly astringent in nature, it is also recommended for diarrhoea, particularly in children.

On a psychological level, neroli's calming effect on the Heart and Mind *(Shen)* associate it mainly with the Fire Element. The oil's delicately rich, floral sweetness is both soothing and euphoric, while its bitter note is at the same time "grounding".

Neroli is ideal for the emotionally intense, sometimes unstable, individual who is easily alarmed and agitated. Due to their heightened sensitivity and response to stress, they can soon become emotionally exhausted, and tend to feel depressed as a result. If, in addition, there is unexpressed anger, or feelings of unconscious resentment, depression may turn to a sense of despair, deep and all-encompassing. Neroli oil instils both comfort and strength, and assists in the release of repressed emotions – through relaxing and reuniting our solar and lunar (conscious and subconscious worlds).

Described as both sensual and spiritual, neroli helps to re-establish the links between a disconnected body and mind. If, for example, nervous depression quells sexual desire, neroli promotes both sensual ease and a feeling of emotional harmony. If, on the other hand, disturbing emotions have been pushed below consciousness, and "somatized" in the body as spasm and pain, neroli paves the way for their gradual release, easing the depression borne of denial. In this way, neroli oil may be considered for any deep emotional pain that robs us of hope and joy.

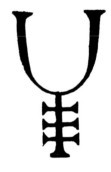

TO AMALGAMATE
The medieval alchemical symbol "to amalgamate" signifies neroli oil's emotionally unifying and harmonizing effects.

Orange

ease ∅ adaptability ∅ optimism

The name "orange" is derived from the Sanskrit for the fruit, *naranj*. Sweet orange oil is extracted through cold expression from the rind of the fruit of *Citrus sinensis*, the sweet orange tree. The *Citrus* genus includes a wide variety of evergreen and semi-evergreen trees and shrubs known principally for their succulent fruit. The forebear of all present-day varieties was most likely the bitter orange *(Citrus aurantium var. amara)*, larger and more hardy than sweet orange. Mandarin *(Citrus reticulata)* is smaller and more spreading than both the sweet and bitter orange trees, with smaller leaves and a more delicately scented peel.

Originating in Asia, the sweet orange was brought to Europe in 1520 by Portuguese explorers returning from southern China, shortly after they had occupied Macao. It thus became known as the "Portugal orange". Along with the lemon, it was introduced to the New World by Columbus, and was grown in both the West Indies and Florida. The largest producers of the essential oil are Brazil, California, Israel, and Florida.

The therapeutic value of the orange was first recognized in Ancient China, where the dried peel has for centuries been an important part of traditional Chinese medicine. Although both ripe and unripe fruits are used, it is the rind of the unripe bitter orange *(zhi shi)* which is of greatest value medicinally – primarily to stimulate the digestion and relieve spasm. It is also a traditional Chinese symbol of good luck and prosperity. In 18th-century Europe, oranges gained a reputation for alleviating nervous disorders, heart problems, colic, asthma, and melancholy.

From an energetic perspective, the principal value of sweet orange oil, like those of bergamot and mandarin, lies in its ability to unblock and circulate stagnant *Qi-energy*, mainly when it accumulates in the Liver, Stomach, and intestines.

Sweet orange is therefore one of the best all-round essential oils for the digestive system. Combining a tonic effect on the Stomach with its ability to circulate *Qi*, the oil is invested with distinct antispasmodic and carminative properties

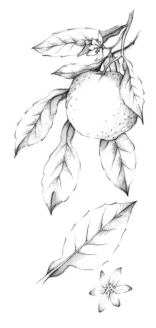

ORANGE, SWEET
Citrus sinensis
FAMILY: *Rutaceae*
PARTS USED: *The rind*
AROMA: *Warm, fresh, citrus & sweet*
ENERGY: *Neutral temperature/neutral moisture*
MAIN ELEMENT: *Wood*
PROPERTIES: *Anti-infectious, antispasmodic, calmative, carminative, cholagogic, digestive stimulant, hepatic stimulant, stomachic*
SAFETY DATA: *Non-toxic; non-irritant*

suitable for abdominal distention and pain, poor appetite, indigestion, flatulence, nausea and vomiting. It can also be effective for constipation and irritable bowel.

Much of the benefit that sweet orange oil can bring depends, in addition, upon its action on the Liver, the organ responsible for ensuring the smooth flow of *Qi-energy*. An hepatic stimulant and cholagogue, the oil not only encourages the flow of bile – improving the digestion of fats – but in addition alleviates general symptoms of stagnant *Liver-Qi*. These include nauseous headaches, tension, and insomnia.

Like bergamot and mandarin, the oil's relaxing, *Qi*-moving and sour qualities all relate it to the Wood Element. Whenever there is an excessive build-up of stress and frustration, the *Qi* becomes blocked and stagnates, causing a disharmony within Liver and a constriction of the Ethereal Soul *(Hun)*. Sweet orange oil helps to move stagnant *Qi* and ease tension and frustration. Its warm, sunny, sweet aroma conveys joy and positivity, dispersing the moodiness and irritability that takes hold when *Qi-energy* stagnates.

More specifically, sweet orange oil is ideally suited to the efficient, hard-working individual who strives for perfection and achievement, but who has little tolerance for mishaps and mistakes. Excellent planners who find it difficult to delegate, they become tense and irritable because they "try too hard". This very tension – and a reluctance to call upon others' help and advice – often seems to invite the very problems they seek to avoid. Ultimately, they come to expect that "things are bound to go wrong".

Sweet orange oil helps us to take a more relaxed approach, encouraging adaptability and the smooth handling of events. Associated with Jupiter, the planet of optimism, it also instils a more positive attitude, and a philosophical view of difficulties. By conveying an easy-going, skilful approach to life, the oil truly embodies "good luck".

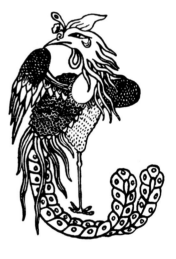

THE PHOENIX
The presentation of oranges at the Chinese New Year betokens the wish for happiness and prosperity during the ensuing twelve months. Honoured as the "Emperor" of birds, the mythical phoenix, too, is a symbol of abundance and good fortune.

Palmarosa

secure Ø fluid Ø adaptable

Palmarosa is a wild herbaceous plant, growing to a height of three metres (nine feet), with long slender stems, fragrant grassy leaves, and flowers in terminal clusters. The flowers turn from a bluish-white colour to dark red as they mature. Palmarosa is a member of the *Cymbopogon* (formerly *Andropogon*) genus of aromatic tropical grasses that includes lemongrass and citronella.

Native to the Indian subcontinent, the grass is cultivated extensively in Madagascar, India, Brazil, and the Comoro Islands. *Cymbopogon martinii* occurs in two varieties: *motia* and *sofia*. Sofia, or "gingergrass", grows best at lower altitudes and in moist and poorly drained soil – in valleys or forests kept humid by rain and fog. The *motia* variety (palmarosa) prefers a *dry*, well-drained soil on sunny mountain slopes and forest clearings, and yields a finer, commercially more important, essential oil. Known as *rosha* in India, palmarosa grass grows wild from the Ganges River to Afghanistan.

Essential oil of palmarosa has been distilled since the 18th century. Under the name of "Indian" or "Turkish geranium oil", it was shipped from Bombay to Constantinople and Bulgaria, where it was used to adulterate rose oil. Although Indian palmarosa continues to be produced in large quantities, it is the Madagascan oil that is now reputedly the finest. Commercially, the oil is used as a fragrance in soaps, perfumes, and cosmetics, as well as to flavour tobacco.

Featured in the Indian *Materia Medica*, both the essential oil and dried herb of palmarosa are employed in Ayurveda (traditional Indian medicine). The oil is recommended for neuralgia, lumbago, sciatica, and rheumatic pain, while the herb is used to treat fevers, dyspepsia, and colitis. It is also mentioned for hair loss. In terms of Oriental medicine, palmarosa oil is *cool* and *moist* in energy. Like rose and geranium, it clears *heat* and strengthens the *yin-energy* – the body's calming, moistening functions.

Palmarosa oil's most common application is in the treatment of skin problems and in skin care generally. Its ability to tonify the *yin* gives it an excellent hydrating property,

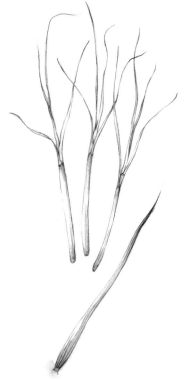

PALMAROSA
Cymbopogon martinii var. motia
FAMILY: *Gramineae (Poaceae)*
PARTS USED: *The grass*
AROMA: *Soft, fresh, citrus, green & rose-like*
ENERGY: *Cool & moist*
MAIN ELEMENT: *Fire*
PROPERTIES: *Antibacterial, antidepressive, anti-infectious, antifungal, anti-inflammatory, antiviral, astringent (mild), calmative, cardiotonic, cellular regenerator, febrifuge, neurotonic, uterine tonic*
SAFETY DATA: *Non-toxic; non-irritant*

helpful for dry, undernourished skin conditions. On the other hand, its cooling, anti-inflammatory nature makes it applicable for dermatitis, eczema, and psoriasis; while the oil's antibacterial, -viral, and -fungal properties make it indicated for a wide range of skin infections, including boils, shingles, and mycosis (fungal infections).

Combined with lavender, tea tree, and geranium oils, palmarosa can also help to clear genito-urinary infections such as cystitis, urethritis, and vaginitis.

A cardiotonic and nervous relaxant, palmarosa oil helps to stabilize both the Heart and nervous system. Reinforcing the *Heart-yin* and calming the Mind *(Shen)*, it is indicated for palpitations, restlessness, insomnia, and anxiety. Palmarosa is particularly good for *hot* conditions where there is tension and exhaustion.

The long stem of this aromatic grass bespeaks of the principal of *movement*: its xylem tissue transporting water and nutrients from the roots to the plant's aerial parts; its phloem tissue conveying nutrients manufactured in the leaves to other parts. At the same time, stem tissues are also used for water and food *storage* – a function that is *yin* in nature.

Conveying a sense of both movement and containment, palmarosa oil on an emotional level encourages both free-flowing adaptability and a feeling of security. The lemony rose-like softness of its aroma is both soothing and astringent, dispersing and gathering. Like rose oil, it centres and comforts the Heart and Mind *(Shen)*, and like lemon, clears away oppression.

Palmarosa oil is suited to individuals who suffer from nervousness and insecurity, but who, in addition, cannot abide change, and the frequent absence of intimate loved ones. They therefore have a tendency to be clinging, possessive, or jealous, finding it hard to "let go" of those they love.

THE HEART CHAKRA
This eightfold Yantra – a yogic visualization tool – is used to restore balance to the Heart Chakra, the vital centre located in the chest. It is a central focus for the subtle, emotionally soothing action of palmarosa oil.

Patchouli

earthing ◊ arousing ◊ enriching

Patchouli is a bushy perennial herb, growing to a height of one metre (three feet), with a sturdy stem, soft, hairy leaves, and flowers in terminal spikes, white with a tinge of mauve. Native to Southeast Asia, the shrub grows wild in Sumatra and Java between altitudes of 900 and 1,800 metres (3,000 and 6,000 feet).

As a crop, it is cut two to three times per year, the best quality being harvested in the wet season. The strongly scented leaves are picked by hand, and are dried for three days before distillation. Most of the world's supply of patchouli oil comes from Indonesia, though China, Malaysia, and India are also producers.

The popular name of the oil is derived from the Hindustan *pacholi*, as it was used in the 19th century to scent Indian fabrics and shawls. French garment manufacturers were obliged to scent their homespun imitations with patchouli oil in order to ensure their saleability. With its persistent base-note aroma, patchouli oil is an excellent natural fixative, and plays an important role within perfumery. It is one of the few essential oils with the distinction of improving with age.

Patchouli has for centuries been part of the traditional systems of medicine in Malaysia, China, and Japan. Attributed with anti-inflammatory and astringent properties, it is indicated for dermatitis, enteritis, and diarrhoea. As an antiseptic fumigant and rubbing oil, it was used to prevent the spread of fevers and epidemics, and was thought to strengthen the immune system. It is also considered to be an effective insecticide, and continues to be one of the most important remedies for snake and insect bites.

From an energetic perspective, patchouli oil, like jasmine, is *warm* in nature and yet anti-inflammatory in action. It combines a calmative property with a gently stimulating one, a synergistic effect that results in a feeling of uplift.

A valuable skin remedy, patchouli oil's antiseptic and emollient properties combine to make it applicable for a wide variety of dermal disorders. As a regenerator of the tissues, it helps to rejuvenate the skin when it is cracked and sore, and

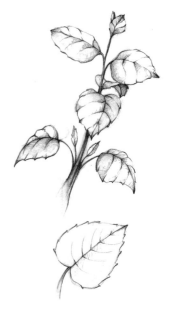

PATCHOULI
Pogostemon cablin
FAMILY: *Labiatae (Lamiaceae)*
PARTS USED: *The young leaves and shoots*
AROMA: *Sweet, warm, earthy, musky, and spicy*
ENERGY: *Neutral temperature/dry*
MAIN ELEMENT: *Earth (& Fire)*
PROPERTIES: *Antibacterial, anti-infectious, anti-inflammatory, antifungal, cicatrisant, decongestant, digestive stimulant, febrifuge, immune tonic, insect repellent, phlebotonic, sexual tonic, stomachic, tissue regenerator*
SAFETY DATA: *Non-toxic; non-irritant*

is therefore useful for eczema. As an antibacterial and anti-viral essential oil, it may also be used for acne, impetigo, and herpes. Combined with oils of cypress and geranium, patchouli may be used, in addition, as a vascular deconges-tant and astringent phlebotonic, suitable for haemorrhoids and varicose veins.

However, patchouli oil's most valuable therapeutic use is mainly energetic and psychological. Earthy, *warm,* and sweet, it may be used for people with a deficiency of *Qi-energy* in the Spleen-pancreas, and who, as a result, suffer from fatigue, loose stools, and abdominal distention. The oil is particularly relevant for conditions of weak immunity, where overwork and chronic anxiety have left the person prone to infection.

Psychologically, patchouli oil works through harmonizing the Element Earth and the Intellect *(Yi),* grounding and stabilizing the mind when overthinking and worry develop. It is also good for those who, due to excessive mental activity and nervous strain, feel "out of touch" with their body and their sensuality. Rich and musky, patchouli oil in this respect is a relaxing aphrodisiac, similar in action to jasmine and ylang ylang. It may be helpful for those with impotence, frigidity, and sexual anxiety.

Like basil and damiana, patchouli oil combines an aphrodisiac effect with an antidepressive one. Quelling an overactive intellect and gently stimulating the senses, the oil is able to uplift the Mind *(Shen),* and through its spicy warmth gladden and inspire.

Patchouli oil is ideally suited to the mentally active and tense individual who easily feels divorced from both sensual pleasure and creative expression. It may be used, therefore, not only to arouse and uplift, but to facilitate the activity of the fertile imagination, reawakening the urge to "conceive".

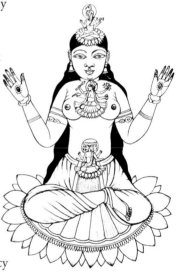

THE TRIAD OF FORCES
Depicted here are the three prin-cipal forces at work within the subtle body. Located at the navel centre is the creative force of Brahma; at the heart is the balanc-ing, preserving influence of Vishnu; and at the crown, the transcenden-tal power of Shiva. Patchouli oil affects, and helps to harmonize, all three forces.

Peppermint

attentive ∅ tolerant ∅ visionary

Peppermint is a perennial herb, growing to a height of 30 to 100 centimetres (11 to 39 inches), with sharply toothed, lanceolate leaves and white, occasionally mauve, flowers. *Mentha piperita* belongs to a genus consisting of some 20 varieties and hybrids, all containing essential oil in their stems and leaves. Native to the Mediterranean and western Asia, mints now grow in temperate regions the world over.

Among the many types of mint cultivated, peppermint is the most commercially and medicinally important. Other varieties of mint include spearmint *(Mentha spicata)*, water mint *(Mentha aquatica)*, field mint *(Mentha arvensis)*, and bergamot mint *(Mentha x citrata)*. Peppermint is thought to be a hybrid between spearmint and water mint.

According to hieroglyphics found in the temple of Edfu, mint was used by the Ancient Egyptians as a ritual perfume, and was an ingredient of the sacred incense *kyphi*. In Ancient Greece and Rome, mint was an everyday part of life, used to scent bath water and, in powdered form, bedding. Celebrated both as a carminative and tonic of the nerves, Pliny declared that the "very smell of it alone recovers and refreshes the spirit". Peppermint essential oil was used as early as the 14th century to whiten teeth, and later to mask the smell of tobacco.

The name of the genus is thought to derive from the Greek myth in which Minthe, a nymph pursued by Pluto, was changed by the jealous Persephone into a sweet-smelling herb. Other sources report that *Mentha* is derived from the Latin *mente*, meaning "thought".

The pungent, stimulating nature of peppermint produces, in the first instance, a warming effect on the body. However, the effect of the essential oil is ultimately cooling and refreshing, and is for this reason better suited to relieving conditions of a *hot* nature. Energetically *cool* and *dry*, peppermint oil circulates *Qi-energy*, clears *hot phlegm*, and stimulates the nerves and brain. It also has an anti-infectious action.

In this regard, peppermint oil is useful for colds and influenza characterized by strong fever, sore throat, and

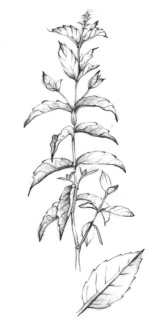

PEPPERMINT *Mentha piperita*
FAMILY: *Labiatae (Lamiaceae)*
PART USED: *The leaf*
AROMA: *Fresh, cool, pungent & sweet; clean & minty*
ENERGY: *Cool & dry*
MAIN ELEMENT: *Earth & Wood*
PROPERTIES: *Analgesic, antibacterial, anticatarrhal, antifungal, anti-infectious, anti-inflammatory, antispasmodic, antiviral, carminative, cephalic, choleretic, digestive stimulant, expectorant, febrifuge, hepatic stimulant, insect repellent*
SAFETY DATA: *Do not use in pregnancy or while breast-feeding, or on children under 2 yrs. Avoid using on individuals with epilepsy, fever, or heart disease. Do not use at more than 2% dilution, or more than 1ml per 24 hours (adult)*

headache. Here, it may be diluted in a base oil together with cypress, eucalyptus, and lemon oils, and applied to the shoulders, neck, and temples. A mild expectorant, it will also benefit respiratory conditions involving sticky, yellow mucus, or *hot phlegm*. It may therefore be used as an adjunctive remedy for chronic bronchitis and bronchial asthma, especially where the digestion is weak.

Stimulating the flow of *Qi-energy* in the Stomach and intestines, peppermint is one of the most effective oils for the digestive system, relieving dyspepsia, nausea, epigastric distention, and flatulence. The oil's antispasmodic and anti-inflammatory actions are also of benefit for intestinal colic, mucous colitis, and hepatitis.

Peppermint oil's antispasmodic nature rests partly in its action on the nervous system. Fresh and pungent in nature, it stimulates and awakens both the nerves and brain, enhancing concentration and study. While not a major tonic for chronic nervous debility, it is nonetheless useful for mental fatigue, especially where an immediate effect is required.

Invigorating the mind and stimulating the Stomach, peppermint oil has a direct action on the Intellect *(Yi)* and on the Earth Element. While the oil enhances concentration and absorption on one level, it works on another level to facilitate the digestion of new ideas and impressions. Acting on our psychological "stomach", peppermint oil is conducive not only to study and learning, but to developing emotional tolerance. We can think of it for those states characterized by the phrase, "That's something I just can't stomach!"

John Gerard, in 1597, believed that "the savour or smell of the water mint rejoiceth the heart of a man". Traditionally classified as a Visionary Herb, mint was thought not only to uplift the Spirit, but to bring dreams of prophecy. Clearly, peppermint oil enhances our receptive capacities on both mental and spiritual levels, and like clary sage and laurel, benefits those in need of inspiration and insight.

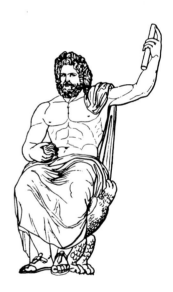

ZEUS, GOD OF HEAVEN
Mint was dedicated by the Ancient Greeks to Zeus, the king of the gods. As lord of the sky and of lightning, Zeus reflects peppermint oil's visionary potential – its ability to stimulate both clarity of mind and flashes of intuition.

$\mathcal{P}$ine

distinct self-identity Ø vibrant self-image

Scots pine is a tall evergreen tree, growing to a height of
40 metres (131 feet), with deeply fissured, reddish-brown
bark, pairs of stiff blue-green needles, and pointed brown
cones. The *Pinus* genus consists of more than 100 species of
coniferous trees, all producing a resin from which turpentine
oil can be extracted. The Scots or Norway pine *(Pinus
sylvestris)* is the most widespread variety, as well as the safest
and most useful therapeutically – though maritime pine
(Pinus pinaster) and terebinth *(Pinus mugo)* are also important. Native to northern Europe and Russia, Scots pine now
grows abundantly in North America as well. The needles,
young branches, and cones can all be used in the distillation
process, though the best quality essential oil is extracted from
the needles alone.

The straight, unbranched cylindrical trunks of the pine
have for centuries furnished a valuable timber, and were once
the favourite source of masts for sailing ships. The kernels
were eaten by the Ancient Egyptians, who added them to
bread, while the young tops were used by the American
Indians to prevent scurvy. They would also burn twigs with
cedar and juniper for the ritual smudging of the sweat lodge,
in order to purify the Spirit. Like the Swiss, they used the
dried needles to stuff their mattresses.

Both Dioscorides and Galen recommended the cones,
especially when boiled with horehound and honey, for "an
old cough" and "the cleansing of the chest and lungs". It later
became traditional practice to add the young macerated
shoots to the bath, to relieve both rheumatic pain and nervous exhaustion.

In terms of Oriental medicine, pine oil is *warm* and *dry*,
and tonifies *Qi-energy*. Expectorant, balsamic, and antiseptic,
it is indicated, in particular, for a wide variety of pulmonary
complaints, though it also benefits conditions such as
rheumatism.

Pine is one of the best essential oils to clear *cold phlegm*
from the Lungs, and to fight respiratory tract infections.
It can be used for sinus and bronchial congestion, coughs,

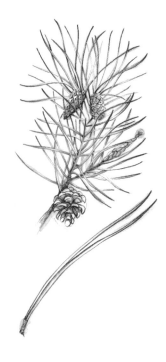

Scots Pine
Pinus sylvestris
Family: *Pinaceae*
Parts used: *The needles*
Aroma: *Strong, fresh, coniferous,
balsamic & woody*
Energy: *Warm & dry*
Main element: *Metal*
Properties: *Analgesic, anti-
bacterial, anti-infectious, anti-
inflammatory, antirheumatic,
balsamic, decongestant, expecto-
rant, hypertensive, litholytic,
neurotonic, rubefacient*
Safety data: *Non-toxic;
non-irritant*

asthma, and bronchitis. Combined with common thyme, eucalyptus, and tea tree, it is also good for colds and influenza characterized by chills, fatigue, and clear or whitish catarrh.

With regards to the genito-urinary system, pine oil's antiseptic and anti-inflammatory properties may be applied to conditions such as cystitis and pyelitis. By stimulating the Kidneys and reducing uric acid in the blood, this soothing, balsamic oil can also relieve rheumatic pain and arthritis.

A tonic of the Lungs, Kidneys, and nerves, pine ranks alongside rosemary and thyme as one of the most effective oils for fatigue and nervous debility. It is appropriate, in particular, for those in whom exhaustion is coupled with shallow breathing, a wheezy chest, and lower backache.

In line with its energetic effect, pine oil is psychologically fortifying. Its fresh, pungent, "aerial" aroma, and its pronounced action on the Lungs, relate it, in the main, to the Metal Element. Invigorating the Bodily Soul *(P'o)* – the source of our "vital spirit" – pine oil "opens the chest", instils positivity and helps to restore self-confidence. Like essential oils of hyssop and thyme, it disperses melancholy and counteracts pessimism, working to reawaken our instinctive connection to life.

On a more subtle level, it was described by Dr Edward Bach as being indicated "for those who blame themselves", who feel responsible not just for their own actions but for the mistakes and sufferings of others. A Herb of Protection, pine is indicated for the type of Metal Element imbalance where there is a weakness of "boundary" and of self-identity – where one cannot distinguish others' responsibilities from one's own. Unable to transmute the forces of their environment, such an individual will tend to turn inward, feeling helpless and unworthy.

Restoring emotional positivity and "boundary", as well as our ability to "process" experience, pine works to dissipate both a negative self-image and feelings of remorse, replacing undue guilt with forgiveness and self-acceptance.

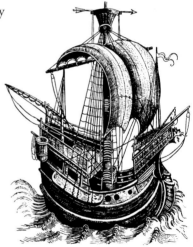

THE SHIP'S MAST
The tall, upright, and unbranched trunk of the Scots pine made it a highly valued source of wood for the masts of sailing ships.

Rose

love Ø trust Ø self-acceptance

The damask rose *(Rosa damascena)* is a hardy, deciduous, bushy shrub with a height and spread of up to two metres (six feet). It has grey-green foliage and fragrant double flowers, pink in bud and fading to almost white. Most *Rosa damascena* is cultivated in the Balkan mountains of southern Bulgaria, in the Valley of the Roses.

Originating from Asia, there are some 250 different species of rose, and over 10,000 different hybrid varieties. Among the 30 of these described as "odorata", only three are commonly distilled for their perfume: French rose *(Rosa gallica)*, cabbage rose *(Rosa centifolia)*, and damask rose *(Rosa damascena)*. It is the Bulgarian damask rose, cultivated since the 16th century, which is considered to produce the finest quality distilled essence, or "otto". Most rose oil produced in France is extracted by solvents from cabbage rose, to produce an "absolute". Because it requires as many as 60,000 roses (57kg/120lb) to make 28g (1oz) of rose otto, the absolute is significantly cheaper, and is therefore used by the perfumery industry. Not a true essential oil, the absolute is generally not recommended for therapeutic use, as toxic traces of the solvents remain.

Rose was called "the queen of flowers" by the Greek poet Sappho. The gentle, exquisite sweetness of its aroma, together with its considerable therapeutic value, ensured its special place in the medicine and perfumery of the Ancient Persian, Egyptian, Indian, Greek, and Roman civilizations. It is no less revered today.

The word *rosa* is derived from the Greek word *rodon*, meaning "red". The crimson colour of the rose was said to come from the blood of Adonis, the youthful vegetation god.

In terms of Oriental medicine, rose is *cool* and *moist* in nature, clears *heat* and inflammation, and helps to restore the body's *yin* energy. It is generally indicated for inflamed, toxic and infectious conditions, and for anxiety and depression.

Cooling and regulating the Liver, rose oil is indicated for *hot*, stagnant conditions that result in tension, irritability, headache, and constipation. It can improve the flow of bile,

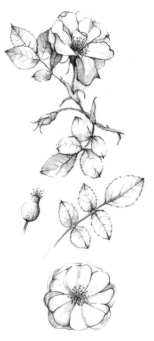

ROSE
Rosa damascena
FAMILY: *Rosaceae*
PART USED: *The flowering tops*
AROMA: *Rich & floral; soft & sweet; slightly sour & astringent*
ENERGY: *Cool & moist*
MAIN ELEMENT: *Fire*
PROPERTIES: *Antibacterial, antidepressive, anti-infectious, anti-inflammatory, astringent, calmative, choleretic, cicatrisant, haemostatic, neurotonic, sexual tonic, general tonic, uterine tonic*
SAFETY DATA: *Non-toxic; non-irritant*

reduce nausea, and help to relieve cholecystitis. Conditions of stagnant *Qi-energy* and *blood* that result in irregular or painful menstruation will also benefit from rose oil. Long considered a tonic of the uterus, its astringent and haemostatic actions make it indicated for excessive menstrual bleeding – especially combined with oils of cypress and geranium.

Rose oil is one of the most suitable ingredients of ointments and lotions for the skin, particularly when it is inflamed or dehydrated, or afflicted by rashes or boils. Rosewater, too, is excellent for soothing and toning skin which is sensitive and dry.

A gentle tonic of the Heart, the key to rose's psychological properties lie mainly in its effect on the Mind *(Shen)*, the centre of our emotional being. Rose oil calms and yet supports the Heart, helping to nourish the *Heart-yin* and restore a sense of well-being. It is of benefit for nervous anxiety, insomnia, and palpitations.

On a more subtle level, the power of rose may be symbolized by its traditional classification as a Herb of Love. Sacred to Aphrodite, Greek goddess of love, beauty, and fertility, the enticing floral sensuality of rose oil has made it a renowned aphrodisiac. At the same time, the damask rose is the Holy Rose, a symbol of God's love for the world. It is often shown surrounding the Virgin, as when she appeared to St Bernadette at Lourdes.

The compassion of the flower is revealed through its ability to heal emotional wounds. When rejection or loss has injured our capacity for self-love and -nurturing, rose oil brings a sweet, gentle comfort, binding the heart-strings of the Mind *(Shen)*. Bringing warmth to a soul grown cold through abuse or hurt, rose oil can touch the deepest despair, restoring the trust that makes it possible to love again.

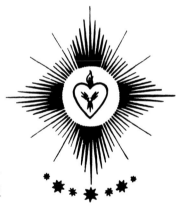

THE RADIANT HEART
This early Christian heart symbol is representative of faith, hope, and love – each of which rose oil seeks to restore to the centre of one's being.

Rosemary

self-identity ∅ dedication ∅ destiny

Rosemary is an evergreen perennial shrub, growing to a height of 80 to 180 centimetres (31 to 50 inches), with leathery, needle-like, silver-green leaves and small, tubular, pale-blue flowers. Originating in the Mediterranean, the herb now grows throughout Europe, North Africa, the Middle East, and California. The name "Rosemary" is derived from the Latin *ros marinus*, meaning "rose of the sea".

Rosemary is one of the most strongly aromatic and widely used of medicinal plants. In Ancient Egypt, the sprigs were burnt as a ritual incense, and placed in the tombs of the pharaohs to help them recall their former life. To the Ancient Greeks and Romans the plant was sacred, symbolic of loyalty, death, and remembrance, as well as scholarly learning. At weddings and important occasions, wherever solemn vows were made, garlands and headdresses of rosemary were worn, as an emblem of trust and constancy. This tradition continued for centuries in Europe, where in wealthy homes sprigs of gilded rosemary would be presented to guests as a token of love and friendship.

At funerals, rosemary was burnt as an incense, in respect and memory of the dead. Valued by the ancients for its power to enhance concentration, its association with remembrance persisted for centuries, the most famous evidence of this being uttered by the tragic Ophelia: "There's rosemary, that's for remembrance".

The plant was also thought to bring good luck, and to impart protection against magic and witchcraft. This would have mirrored the power it was accorded as a medicinal, with the strength both to safeguard against the plague and to reinvigorate health: "Seethe much Rosemary," advised William Langham (1597), "and bathe therein to make thee lusty, lively, joyfull, likeing and youngly".

Essential oil of rosemary was first distilled in the 13th century. One of the most valuable and invigorating of essences, it is an excellent tonic of the body's *yang* energy, able in addition to promote the circulation of both *Qi-energy* and *blood*. *Warm*, pungent, and stimulating, it can help to rectify both

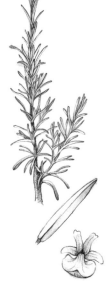

Common Rosemary
Rosmarinus officinalis
Family: *Labiatae (Lamiaceae)*
Part used: *The sprig*
Aroma: *Strong, fresh, camphoraceous, balsamic & slightly woody*
Energy: *Warm & dry*
Main element: *Fire*
Properties: *Antibacterial, anticatarrhal, antifungal, anti-infectious, antirheumatic, antispasmodic, cardiotonic, carminative, cephalic, choleretic, diuretic (mild), emmenagogic, expectorant, hepatic stimulant, hypertensive, litholytic, neurotonic, sexual tonic, general tonic*
Safety data: *Do not use in pregnancy or while breast-feeding, or on children under 2 yrs. Avoid using on individuals with epilepsy or fever. Do not use at more than 2% dilution*

mental and physical malaise. Energizing the *Qi-energy* of the Heart, rosemary oil strengthens the heartbeat and encourages the flow of arterial blood. It is of benefit for cardiac fatigue, palpitations, low blood pressure, and cold hands and feet. As it increases blood supply to the brain, the oil can also be used for poor concentration and nervous debility, and is therefore classified as a *cephalic*.

Moving both the *Qi-energy* and *blood*, rosemary oil is an excellent tonic of the muscles, and is used for muscular stiffness, cramping, and pain. It is also one of the best antirheumatic essential oils, indicated for joint pain of a *cold*, fixed, and cramping nature.

Expectorant in action, rosemary oil may be used for *cold*, catarrhal coughs and bronchitis; and as a carminative and choleretic, it helps to relieve dyspepsia, flatulence, and abdominal distention.

Rosemary was traditionally viewed as an exhilarating herb, naturally ruled by the Sun – astrological symbol of vitality and individuality. A plant that could renew enthusiasm and bolster self-confidence, it was an age-old remedy for apathy and gloom. Rosemary is suited to the cold, debilitated individual who has a poor sense of self-worth and who lacks a strong, healthy ego – an ego that values its place in the world, and goes in pursuit of its own fulfilment. Their tendency to overthink and doubt their every action dilutes their resolve and dampens their "vital fire".

Reinforcing the Heart and empowering the Mind *(Shen)*, rosemary oil helps to boost the confidence and morale of those who lack faith in their own potential. It warms the Spirit and makes it bold.

Although not a tender, enticing essential oil like rose or neroli, rosemary nonetheless inspires, through its sweet, reviving freshness, the fervent faith and joy of love. Like caraway oil, it enhances the spiritual dedication of love rather than the experience of romantic ecstasy. And as a Herb of Remembrance, it helps us not only to recall loved ones but to remember our own true path.

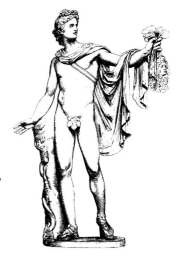

APOLLO, GOD OF LIGHT
Rosemary was dedicated by the Ancient Greeks to the solar deity of Apollo, the god of medicine, music, poetry, and prophecy. Apollo is an archetypal symbol of the heroic side of human nature, and of the same power of conscious self-determination as brought to the fore by rosemary oil.

Sandalwood

stillness ∅ unity ∅ being

Sandalwood is a parasitic evergreen tree, growing to a height of nine metres (29 feet), with leathery leaves and small purple flowers. The essential oil is extracted from the tree's heartwood. Native to southern Asia, most of the world's *Santalum album* is grown in the Mysore region of eastern India. Other varieties such as *Santalum rubrum* grow in Australia and the Pacific Islands, but are without the medicinal value of *Santalum album.*

The long history of sandalwood in the cultural and spiritual life of Asia cannot be overstated. The wood was carved into furniture, temples, and religious icons, is burned as an incense in Buddhist and Hindu temples, and retains an important place in Ayurvedic, Tibetan, and traditional Chinese medicines. As a Funeral Herb, it is used to anoint and embalm the dead, and to carry the soul into the next life. For the yogi it is believed to encourage the meditative state and to enhance devotion to God.

In Ayurvedic (traditional Indian) medicine sandalwood is valued for its anti-inflammatory, antifebrile, and anti-infectious properties. Frequently applied as a paste for inflamed skin, it is classified according to Ayurveda as a medicinal for conditions of *pitta*, or *fire.*

Cool and decongesting, sandalwood oil is primarily indicated for problems of a *hot*, inflammatory, and catarrhal nature, particularly where the intestines, genito-urinary system and lungs are involved. As a gently sedating analgesic, it also helps to relieve pain.

Sandalwood oil is outstanding for intestinal and genito-urinary conditions that require a cooling, astringent effect – as in cases of "burning" diarrhoea, mucous colitis, and vaginal discharge of a yellowish colour. Mildly anti-infectious, it may also be combined with lavender, tea tree, and geranium oils as part of an ointment for *hot*, "burning" cystitis.

Sandalwood oil, in addition, is useful for respiratory mucus and infection – especially when a soothing, demulcent effect is required. In cases of bronchitis involving a "thick", harsh and painful cough, sandalwood may be combined with oils

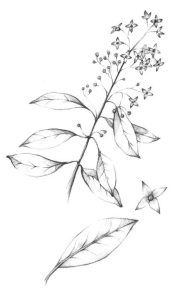

SANDALWOOD
Santalum album
FAMILY: *Santalaceae*
PART USED: *The heartwood*
AROMA: *Woody, balsamic, sweet & slightly musky*
ENERGY: *Cool & moist*
MAIN ELEMENT: *Earth (& Water)*
PROPERTIES: *Antidepressive, antifungal, anti-inflammatory, anti-infectious, astringent, expectorant, haemostatic, calmative, cardiotonic, carminative, lymphatic decongestant, sexual tonic, general tonic*
SAFETY DATA: *Non-toxic; non-irritant*

of eucalyptus and geranium. In very low dilution it may also be employed as a gargle for sore throats.

An excellent oil for the skin, sandalwood may be used for dryness, irritation, itching, and inflammation, and is helpful for both eczema and psoriasis.

Sandalwood oil's influence on the mind and Spirit relate at a basic level to its cooling, calming, and toning effect on the nervous system. It may be used effectively for *hot*, agitated emotional states that lead to headache, insomnia, and nervous exhaustion.

Sandalwood's subtle properties are equally reflected in its traditional use as an aid to meditation, prayer, and spiritual practice generally. Its "divinely sweet", softly balsamic, base-note characteristics evoke the Element Earth at its most sensual yet deeply tranquil. Clarifying and stilling the mind – and refreshing an over-heated body – sandalwood oil reconnects us to our primordial sense of being. Diminishing the tyranny of the intellect, of the incessant need to overthink, it instils in its place an experience of inner unity – a state where body, mind, and Spirit can re-align as one.

The paradox of sandalwood is that while it can encourage states of "higher" consciousness, it does so not through any sort of other-worldly effect but by bringing us back to our essential self, to a more immediate awareness of palpable life itself. It is therefore indicated for states of obsessive worry, and for worldly "over-attachment". Whenever we over-invest in seeing specific outcomes to our efforts – especially out of a neurotic need for security – sandalwood oil helps to re-establish an acceptance of reality as it is.

By quelling the mind as an incessant tool of analysis and expectation, sandalwood actually frees it as a creative source, always present in the here and now. It is perhaps for this reason that it has been associated, in terms of the symbolism of the Tarot, with the Empress – the universal womb in which all manifestation is gestated, and the Great Mother of Ideas.

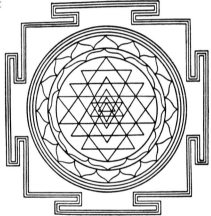

SRI YANTRA
The Sri Yantra is the most well-known and powerful of all yogic Yantras – visual tools of spiritual transformation. Through its combination of upward-pointing Shiva, and downward-pointing Shakti, triangles, it reflects the ability of sandalwood oil to integrate the Spirit with the senses.

Spikenard

stability Ø faith Ø surrender

Spikenard (also called "nard") is a tender aromatic herb, growing to a height of one metre (three feet), with large, lanceolate leaves, small greenish flowers and a fragrant rhizome-root. The rhizome, covered by a tuft of soft, slender, light-brown rootlets, yields the plant's essential oil. A member of the Valerian family, the herb is similar in its aroma and action to Indian valerian *(Valeriana wallachii)*, and indeed is sometimes referred to as "false Indian valerian". Native to the Himalayan mountains, the plant grows wild in Nepal, Bhutan, and Sikkim, at elevations of between 3,000 and 5,000 metres (11,000 and 17,000 feet) – though it is also to be found in China and Japan.

Spikenard is one of the most ancient of aromatics, considered precious to the early Egyptian, Hebrew, and Hindu civilizations for both ritual and medicinal purposes. Mentioned in *The Song of Solomon*, spikenard also appears in *The Gospel According to St John*. Here, the oil is used by Mary Magdalene to anoint Jesus before the Last Supper: "Then took Mary a pound of ointment of spikenard, very costly, and anointed the feet of Jesus, and wiped his feet with her hair; and the house was filled with the odour of the ointment". Like frankincense and myrrh, the association of the herb with Jesus highlights its age-old mystical significance.

Both the female perfumers of Ancient Greece and the *unguentarii* of Rome made use of spikenard in the preparation of *nardinum*, one of the most renowned of scented oils. In his 1st century text, *On Therapeutic Substances*, Dioscorides expressed the classical view of spikenard as a medicinal having "a warming, drying and diuretic faculty", useful for nausea, flatulence, cervicitis, and conjunctivitis. In 1652, Nicholas Culpeper added that it "comforts the brain" and helps "passions and swoonings of the heart".

Indeed, it is mainly used in modern aromatherapy for its regulating action on the nervous system and heart. In terms of Oriental medicine, spikenard oil calms the Heart, stabilizes the Mind *(Shen)* and settles the emotions. Like valerian, it can be used for nervous tension, anxiety, and insomnia,

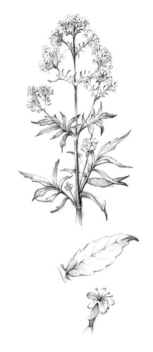

SPIKENARD
Nardostachys jatamansi
FAMILY: *Valerianaceae*
PART USED: *The rhizome and roots*
AROMA: *Warm, earthy, peaty, bittersweet & woody*
ENERGY: *Neutral temperature/dry*
MAIN ELEMENT: *Fire (& Wood)*
PROPERTIES: *Anti-inflammatory, antispasmodic, calmative, cardio-tonic, carminative, digestive stimulant, diuretic (mild), neuro-tonic, phlebotonic*
SAFETY DATA: *Non-toxic; non-irritant*

and for tachycardia and arrhythmia (rapid and irregular heartbeat). Regulating the flow of *Liver-Qi* and of *Qi-energy* in general, spikenard oil has an antispasmodic, digestive action that makes it indicated for nausea, constipation, and intestinal colic. Because it circulates and strengthens *Liver-blood*, the oil is also recommended for haemorrhoids and varicose veins, and for ovarian insufficiency and anaemia.

The *Liver-blood* – the functional relationship between the *blood* and the Liver – relates in addition to the proper nourishment of the skin. By tonifying *Liver-blood* and clearing inflammation, spikenard oil is able to both nourish and soothe the skin, and benefits conditions such as dermatitis and psoriasis.

Just as the energetic actions of spikenard centre on the Heart and Liver, so do the psychological effects of the oil pertain mainly to the Mind *(Shen)* and Ethereal Soul *(Hun)*. Warm and earthy, spikenard oil's calming effect on the Mind helps to soothe the deepest forms of anxiety, and like myrrh, can instill a profound sense of peace. With its added bitter-sweet pungency, it helps, in addition, to release obstruction of *Qi* and *blood*, and so free the Ethereal Soul. Like oil of everlasting, it works to replace despondency and resentment with acceptance and compassion.

Valued as a sacred chrism, spikenard was used as a consecrated oil for monarchs and high initiates. It relates to that eternal part of ourselves that exists beyond the flux of illusion and suffering.

Spikenard oil is therefore indicated for the type of individual who, searching for spiritual certainty, struggles in vain to find the stable ground of faith. Emotional wounds, persistent anxieties, and difficult worldly circumstances can all stand in the way. Nourishing the hope of both heart and soul, spikenard allows us to "surrender", and, through its serenity and earthy humility, conveys the power of devotion to one's chosen path.

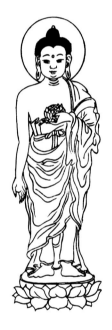

AMIDA BUDDHA
The Amida Buddha has been a popular object of devotion since the 5th century. A symbol of spiritual peace and compassion, his benevolent power to restore faith and tranquillity echoes the qualities of spikenard oil.

Tea Tree

strength Ø resistance Ø confidence

Tea tree is a small tree, growing to a height of seven metres (22 feet), with narrow, soft, alternate leaves and yellowish flowers the shape of bottlebrushes. One of more than 30 species of "paperbark" trees that flourish in Australia, tea tree belongs to the *Melaleuca* genus, and is closely related to *Melaleuca leucadendron* (the source of cajuput oil) and *Melaleuca quinquenervia* (which produces niaouli oil). The name *Melaleuca* comes from the Greek *melas* (black) and *leukos* (white) – referring to the contrast between the dark-green foliage, which appears black, and the loose, paper-thin and very white bark.

Because the water-resistant "paperbark" is so easy to peel off the tree, it was used extensively by the aboriginal peoples of Australia to make small canoes, knife sheaths, and thatching for shelters. The pungent leaves were soaked in hot water and taken as a cure for colds, coughs, and headaches – or they were simply picked from the tree and chewed.

Melaleuca alternifolia thrives in a relatively small area of New South Wales, in swampy low-lying land surrounding flood-prone river systems. Because tea tree favours rather remote wetlands, harvesting the leaves for their oil is difficult.

After landing the H.M.S. Endeavour at Botany Bay in 1770, Captain James Cook and his party came upon a grove of trees thick with sticky, aromatic leaves that they later found made a spicy tea. The "Tea Tree", as it was called by Captain Cook, became a valued bush remedy used by the early European settlers.

However, it was not until after the First World War that serious attention was given to the plant's specific medical uses. In 1923 an Australian government scientist, Dr A. R. Penfold, conducted a study of tea tree essential oil, and discovered it to be 12 times stronger as an antiseptic bactericide than carbolic acid (the current standard). Research continued, and tea tree became recognized, according to the *British Medical Journal* in 1933, as "a powerful disinfectant, non-poisonous and non-irritating". Indeed, among the essential oils valued for their anti-infectious properties, tea tree has

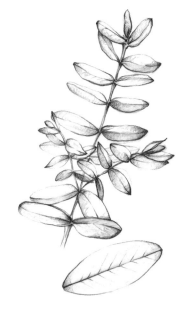

TEA TREE
Melaleuca alternifolia
FAMILY: *Myrtaceae*
PART USED: *The leaf*
AROMA: *Strong, medicinal, camphoraceous, balsamic & bittersweet*
ENERGY: *Warm & dry*
MAIN ELEMENT: *Metal (& Fire)*
PROPERTIES: *Analgesic, antibacterial, antifungal, anti-infectious, antiparasitic, antiviral, balsamic, cardiotonic, cicatrisant, immune tonic, neurotonic, phlebotonic, general tonic, vulnerary*
SAFETY DATA: *Non-toxic; non-irritant*

few rivals. Powerfully antibiotic – literally "against life" – the oil is nevertheless supportive to the life of the body and immune system, and may be safely employed for a wide range of bacterial, viral, and fungal infections. Because tea tree oil strengthens the *Defensive-Qi*, it can be used not only to eradicate harmful pathogens, but to help prevent the recurrence of infection.

The oil may be used for infections that include colds, flu, and bronchitis; sinusitis, otitis and pyorrhoea; candidiasis and viral enteritis; and cystitis and vaginal thrush. Like niaouli oil, it may also be used for bacterial and fungal skin infections, such as impetigo and tinea versicolor.

Tea tree oil is renowned not only for its anti-infectious, immunostimulant action but for its power to reinforce the Lungs, Heart, and nervous system. Like essential oil of common thyme, it will tonify *Qi-energy* in cases of chronic lethargy, shallow breathing, palpitations, and poor circulation. Steadying the nerves and promoting blood-flow to the brain, tea tree oil is also indicated for mental fatigue and nervous debility, especially in people whose immune system is weak.

While immune-related disorders such as myalgic encephelomyelitis (ME) have on occasion been erroneously diagnosed as "depression", there is no doubt that feelings of depression will nevertheless lower one's immunity. In such cases, tea tree is the ideal essential oil to bolster morale as well as resistance.

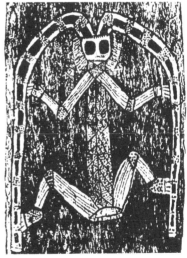

THE LIGHTNING GOD
This aboriginal bark painting of the Lightning God is reminiscent of the lightning-quick force of tea tree oil in combating infection and disease.

Fortifying the Lungs and Bodily Soul *(P'o)* through its camphoraceous pungency, it helps to promote both a positive outlook and the healing instinct. At the same time, its strong, bittersweet spiciness invigorates the Heart and Mind *(Shen)*, uplifting the Spirit and building confidence.

Tea tree oil is of special importance, therefore, to physically delicate individuals who struggle not only with their bodies but with the feelings of victimization and doom that can easily accompany – and exacerbate – chronic ill-health.

Thyme

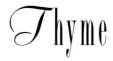

courage ✻ drive ✻ morale

Thyme is a hardy perennial subshrub, growing to a height of 10 to 40 centimetres (three to 15 inches), with hairy, pointed grey-green leaves and small, white-to-lilac flowers. Indigenous to the Mediterranean region of Europe, thyme today grows in temperate regions throughout the world. Spain is the largest producer of the essential oil.

There are more than 300 different varieties of thyme, including garden, or common, thyme *(Thymus vulgaris)*, the less strongly aromatic wild or mother of thyme *(Thymus serpyllum)* and lemon thyme *(Thymus limonum)*, which has a distinct lemony scent.

It is believed that thyme was used by the Ancient Sumerians some 3,500 years ago, most likely burnt as an aromatic fumigant. Calling it *tham*, the Ancient Egyptians employed it in the embalming process, while the Greeks made use of thyme as a culinary herb. They also used it to disinfect the air and so prevent the spread of disease.

So important was the herb's aroma that its name was culled from the Greek *thymon*, meaning "to fumigate". On the other hand, its name has also been linked to the Greek word *thumon*, meaning "courage' – as the plant was associated with bravery. Indeed, Roman soldiers bathed in thyme before entering battle, and in the Middle Ages sprigs of thyme were woven into the scarves of knights departing for the Crusades.

Thyme is one of the most energetically *hot* and invigorating of essential oils, classified by the herbalist John Gerard in 1597 as "hot and dry in the third [or strongest] degree". It is a powerful tonic of the body's *yang* energy, reinforcing the functions of the Lungs, Heart, Kidneys, and nervous system. Strongly antibacterial, the essential oil is indicated for a wide variety of infections.

As a respiratory tonic, antiseptic, and expectorant, essential oil of common thyme may be used for any *cold* condition involving weakness, congestion and/or infection of the Lungs. It will benefit chronic fatigue, shallow breathing, catarrhal coughs, and bronchitis, especially when there is copious, clear or white catarrh. It will also help to relieve

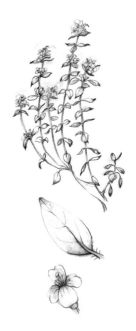

COMMON THYME
Thymus vulgaris thymoliferum
FAMILY: *Labiatae (Lamiaceae)*
PART USED: *The leaves and flowering tops*
AROMA: *Warm, herbaceous, pungent, green & medicinal*
ENERGY: *Hot & dry*
MAIN ELEMENT: *Water & Metal*
PROPERTIES: *Antibacterial, anti-infectious, antiparasitic, antirheumatic, antispasmodic, carminative, cicatrisant, digestive stimulant, diuretic (mild), expectorant, hypertensive, neurotonic, sexual tonic, stomachic, sudorific, general tonic, vermifuge*
SAFETY DATA: *Do not use on children under 2 yrs. Avoid using on individuals with hypersensitive, diseased or damaged skin. Do not use at more than 1% dilution*

colds and influenza with chills and muscular aching.

Like oil of rosemary, thyme tonifies the *yang* energy of the Heart, strengthening the heartbeat and improving circulation. A capillary stimulant, the oil in addition is indicated for anaemia and hair loss. The use of thyme oil will also ease rheumatic pain and arthritis, mainly when characterized by a fixed pain of a contracted or cramping nature.

A digestive stimulate and carminative, thyme oil promotes appetite, eases abdominal distention, and relieves flatulence. Due to its strong antibacterial, antifungal action, it can also help to counteract intestinal putrefaction, gastroenteritis, and candidiasis. It is thyme's anti-infectious property that makes it useful for genito-urinary infections such as cystitis.

That thyme oil is a powerful tonic of the body's dynamic *yang* energy is further reflected in its invigorating mental-emotional effects. Fortifying and uplifting, the oil is a neurotonic, indicated for nervous debility and chronic anxiety. In fact, during the 18th century the herb was included in the French preparation *baume tranquille*, a formula prescribed for nervous disorders. On a more subtle level, the psychological action of thyme is two-fold: stimulating the Lungs, it dispels despondency; energizing the Kidneys, it instils drive.

Thyme's reputation for enlivening the spirits goes back to classical times, and persisted throughout history. A traditional remedy for melancholy, thyme oil's ability to "open the chest" and revive the Bodily Soul *(P'o)* benefits depressive states characterized by withdrawal, pessimism, and self-doubt.

The herb's equally age-old renown for instilling courage and valour reflects its action on the Water Element and the Will *(Zhi)*. In this respect, thyme oil may be used for poor self-confidence, apathy, and fear. Restoring morale at the very deepest level, thyme seeks to imbue both spiritual fortitude and bodily vigour. Whether demoralized, apprehensive, or alienated, we should always consider reaching for thyme's warm and virile strength.

THOR, GOD OF THUNDERSTORMS
Although Thor was regarded as a generous Germanic deity – a gentle giant – he broke into a thunderous rage when provoked. He was the god, therefore, of both fertility and war. With his magic hammer in hand, he makes a fitting symbol of the assertiveness and bravery that oil of thyme imparts.

Vetiver

nourishing Ø restoring Ø reconnecting

Vetiver is a tall, densely tufted perennial grass, two metres (six feet) high, with long, narrow leaves and a mass of fine, spongy rootlets, light yellow to reddish-brown in colour. It is the fragrant rootlets which, washed, dried, and sliced, are steam-distilled for their essential oil, a viscous amber liquid. Together with palmarosa, lemongrass, and citronella, vetiver belongs to the *Gramineae*, or grass, family, the group of plants that provides more edible species (cereal grains included) than all other plant families put together.

In its wild state, vetiver flourishes on the slopes of the Himalayan mountains, and in southern India, Sri Lanka, and Malaysia. The finest-quality vetiver oil, called "Bourbon vetiver", originates from the Réunion Islands, although large quantities are also produced in Haiti and Java.

The common name for the grass comes from its Tamil name, *vetiverr*, meaning "hatcheted up" – a description of the way in which the roots are collected. In Java vetiver is called *akar wangi*, or "fragrant root".

Indeed, it is the rich, earthy fragrance of the root that has for centuries bequeathed it a valued place in Indian households. Woven into heavy blinds and screens, the wiry, fibrous roots darken the windows of homes in the burning noon of summer. Constantly doused with water, the cool, sweet scent of their vapour turns scorching winds that dehydrate into moist and balmy breezes. Because its fragrance repels insects, vetiver fans are cherished by women from India to Java.

An important perfume constituent, the essential oil, like those of sandalwood and patchouli, affords a rich and tenacious base-note characteristic that serves as a fixative for Oriental perfumes. Sanskrit texts refer to its use as an unguent for anointing brides.

An ancient remedy within Ayurveda (traditional Indian medicine), the root and its essential oil are used to alleviate thirst, heatstroke, fevers, and headache. The oil is applied, in addition, as part of a liniment to relieve inflammatory disorders of the joints and skin, and may be used for rheumatoid arthritis and eczema.

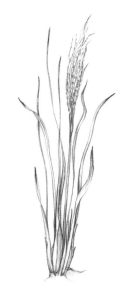

VETIVER
Vetiveria zizanoides
FAMILY: *Gramineae (Poaceae)*
PART USED: *The root*
AROMA: *Sweet & warm; rich & resinous; sightly woody & smoky*
ENERGY: *Cool & moist*
MAIN ELEMENT: *Earth*
PROPERTIES: *Antidepressive, anti-infectious, antirheumatic, antispasmodic, calmative, digestive stimulant, emmenagogic, hepatic stimulant, immune tonic, pancreatic stimulant, phlebotonic, general tonic*
SAFETY DATA: *Non-toxic; non-irritant*

In terms of Oriental medicine, vetiver oil is *cool* and *moist* in energy. It clears *heat*, nourishes, calms, and uplifts. From a vitalistic viewpoint, the roots of any plant are innately nourishing, strengthening, and grounding. Belonging to a family that feeds the world, the roots of vetiver are especially so – a fact reflected in the very richness of the oil.

It is this nurturing quality of the plant that gives it the ability to support the *yin* – the body's restorative, absorptive, anabolic functions. Vetiver oil is for this reason indicated for poor appetite, weight loss, anaemia, and malabsorption. Renewing the strength of the body's connective tissue, it may also be used for both weakness of the joints and dry, undernourished skin. And as a tonic of glands, it is indicated for oestrogen and progesterone insufficiency, and for the premenstrual tension and menopausal problems that can result.

Vetiver's ability to cool and nourish the body is reflected in its actions on a psychological level. Relaxing an overheated, hyperactive mind and nurturing an insecure self-identity, the oil imbues us with the calm, reassuring strength of Mother Earth, and her deep sense of belonging. Whether mentally exhausted from overwork, or out of touch with our body and its needs, vetiver sedates and yet restores us – centres and reconnects us – closing the gap between Spirit and matter.

It is therefore suited to the type of individual who constantly strives for perfection, but who, in the process of pursuing their ideal, loses touch with the ability to absorb and replenish, and are never still enough to let perfection *be*. The uplift that vetiver brings them is one that, paradoxically, comes of travelling *down* – down to that experience where we instinctively rejoice in feeling essentially *real*.

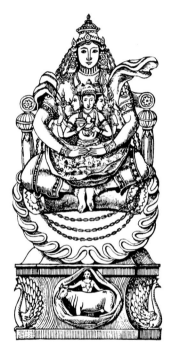

PRAKRITI, THE POWER OF MANIFESTATION
According to the Indian philosophy of Vedanta, Prakriti is a feminine symbol of the universal energy, and of the power of manifestation. Through its capacity to reconnect us to our vital source, vetiver oil instils a sense of her potency.

Yarrow

protecting ∅ mollifying ∅ healing

Yarrow is a perennial creeping herb, growing to a height of 10 to 60 centimetres (three to 23 inches), with erect stems, lace-like leaves divided into feathery leaflets, and a composite head of numerous, tiny, daisy-like flowers, white or pink in colour. Native to Europe, the plant now grows wild in temperate regions throughout the world. Most of the world's yarrow oil is produced in Eastern Europe – in Albania, Hungary, and Bulgaria in particular.

The common name for the plant, "yarrow", is a corruption of its Anglo-Saxon name, *gearwe*, while its specific name, *millefolium*, refers to the many segments of its foliage – the reason it has also been called "milfoil" and "thousand leaf".

However, it is the term given to its generic name, *Achillea*, which is most revealing. Long valued for its wound-healing properties, it was dedicated to Achilles, the wrathful warrior of Homer's *Iliad*. According to legend, Achilles employed the plant during the Trojan war to cure his comrade Telephus of a spear wound. Variously referred to as "soldier's wound-wort", "staunchgrass", and "carpenter's weed", it has been used throughout history as a dependable vulnerary – by the knights of the Crusades and by carpenters for chisel cuts.

The folklore surrounding the plant extended to matters of love and loyalty. Inserted into the nostrils, yarrow was supposed to stop bleeding, but as a test of fidelity, it should ideally cause it: "Yarroway, yarroway, bear a white blow/ If my love love me my nose will bleed now". As a Visionary Herb, it is perhaps best known for providing the stalks used to divine the ancient Chinese Oracle, the *I-Ching*.

According to Oriental medicine, yarrow is *cool* and *dry* in nature, and, like chamomile (another *Compositae* member), is both antispasmodic and anti-inflammatory in action.

As an antispasmodic essential oil, yarrow's ability to stimulate the Liver and regulate the flow of *Qi-energy* make it indicated for indigestion, intestinal colic, irritable bowel, and insufficient bile production. As an analgesic, the oil may be used to break through the *bi*, or "painful obstruction", of sprains, rheumatism, and neuralgia. Emmenagogic in nature,

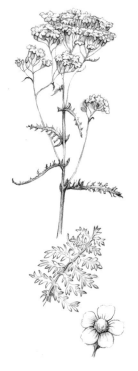

YARROW *Achillea millefolium*
FAMILY: *Compositae (Asteraceae)*
PART USED: *The herb*
AROMA: *Herbaceous, bittersweet, warm & slightly camphoraceous*
ENERGY: *Cool & dry*
MAIN ELEMENT: *Wood (& Metal)*
PROPERTIES: *Analgesic, anticatarrhal, anti-inflammatory, antispasmodic, astringent, choleretic, cicatrisant, digestive stimulant, diuretic (mild), emmenagogic, expectorant, febrifuge, hepatic stimulant, vulnerary*
SAFETY DATA: *Do not use in pregnancy or while breast-feeding, or on children under 2 yrs. Avoid using on individuals with epilepsy or fever. Do not use at more than 2% dilution*

it is also recommended to help alleviate menstrual pain.

An oil that also clears *heat*, yarrow contains the anti-inflammatory molecule chamazulene, helping to make it effective for neuritis, prostatitis, and arthritis. Combined with oils of lavender, cypress, and lemon, it may be used, in addition, for influenza characterized by strong fever and headache. And as a urinary antiseptic, yarrow will help to soothe cystitis and urethritis.

Yarrow oil's action extends to both the Heart and Kidneys: as a gentle cardiotonic, it is indicated for poor circulation and low blood pressure; while as a soothing diuretic, it benefits frequent, scanty urination.

Yarrow's ancient reputation as a "woundwort" relates on a subtle level to its role as a Herb of Protection, as well as its ability to consolidate the "aura" (or personal psychic field). In this regard, yarrow relates to the Metal Element, evident physiologically through its ability to regulate the pores of the skin, our physical boundary.

At the same time, yarrow has a profound action on the Liver and Ethereal Soul *(Hun)*, releasing stagnant *Qi-energy* and the blocked emotions that go with it. Like everlasting oil, it is relevant for deeply repressed anger and embitterment, and echoes symbolically the vengeful wrath of Achilles.

Yarrow oil is most appropriate for those in whom feelings of anger or rage are linked subconsciously with emotional wounding and vulnerability. Easily offended, they tend to strike out furiously at every injury, at all costs determined to keep hurt and "weakness" hidden. On the other hand, the same basic problem may cause them to suppress their feelings of anger and annoyance – submerged as they are by the pain of past wounds.

Yarrow's "visionary" effect on a emotional level is one that helps those in depression release the bitterness of hidden rage; while in those who are habitually defensive and severe, it allows them to tap and relinquish their tears.

THE SWORD IN THE HEART
The sword that pierces the heart is a traditional symbol of deepest sorrow, and of the archetypal Wound. It speaks of the need, as encouraged by yarrow oil, to fully accept pain in order to heal and go beyond it.

Ylang Ylang

relaxing Ø sensualizing Ø euphoric

Ylang ylang is a tropical evergreen tree, reaching a height of twenty metres (65 feet), with large, shiny, ovate leaves and long, narrow, downy flowers that turn from pale green to deep yellow as they mature. It is the freshly picked flowers that contain the essential oil.

Indigenous to Southeast Asia, most of the world's ylang ylang oil is produced in the Comoro Islands, Madagascar, and Réunion. In terms of fragrance quality, there are as many as five grades of ylang ylang, with "Ylang Ylang Extra Superior" being the highest and most expensive. Essential oil of "cananga", the macrophylla variety of *Cananga odorata*, is sometimes sold as ylang ylang *(var. genuina)*, but is harsher and less subtle, though lower in cost.

The name *ylang ylang* comes from the Philippine *alang-ilang*, referring to the flowers that "hang" or "flutter" in the breeze. The islanders would pick the flowers and immerse them in coconut oil, producing a pommade called *boori-boori*. This they used as a body rub to prevent fevers and infections, especially in the rainy season, and to nourish and rejuvenate the skin. The oil was also applied to the hair, to protect it from the salt water of the sea as they swam.

The Indonesians, on the other hand, spread the luxuriant flowers on the marriage bed of newly wedded couples.

Ylang ylang oil has long been one of the most important raw materials within perfumery, its exotic spicy sweetness imparting floral top notes to an otherwise dull and flat composition. Some of the masterpieces of French perfumery have relied on the skilful blending of ylang ylang, rose, bergamot, and vanilla. Ylang ylang's medicinal properties were first recognized at the beginning of the 20th century by the French chemists Garnier and Rechler. Conducting research on the island of Réunion, they discovered the oil to be effective against malaria, typhus, and infections of the intestinal tract. They also noted its calming action on the heart.

In terms of Oriental medicine, it is in fact ylang ylang oil's calming, supportive action on the Heart that accounts for its primary therapeutic action.

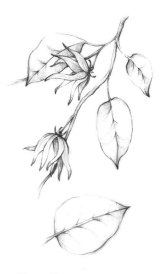

YLANG YLANG
Cananga odorata var. genuina
FAMILY: *Annonaceae*
PART USED: *The flowers*
AROMA: *Floral, sweet, balsamic, heady & slightly spicy*
ENERGY: *Cool & moist*
MAIN ELEMENT: *Fire*
PROPERTIES: *Antidepressive, antidiabetic, anti-infectious, anti-inflammatory, antiparasitic, antispasmodic, calmative, hypotensive, sexual tonic*
SAFETY DATA: *Non-toxic; non-irritant*

Energetically *cool* and *moist*, ylang ylang oil works to clear *heat* from the Heart when severe nervous tension leads to palpitations, hypertension, and tachycardia (rapid heartbeat). Simultaneously harmonizing the Mind *(Shen)* and calming the nervous system, the oil is also known for its ability to "cool down" states of restlessness and agitation, and to help promote sleep. According to Dr Tim Betts of Birmingham University's Neuropsychiatry Clinic, UK, ylang ylang oil can also be effective for controlling epilepsy, especially when smelt before the onset of a seizure: "The majority of patients with epilepsy, given a choice of four or five oils, almost invariably choose ylang ylang". The oil is additionally recommended as a supportive remedy in diabetes, as well as to stimulate the scalp and prevent hair loss.

The aphrodisiac power of ylang ylang oil is inseparable both from its ability to relax and uplift, and from its voluptuous aroma. Indicated for impotence and frigidity, it may be used by people in whom fear, anxiety, and the urge to withdraw have subconsciously blocked their feelings of sexuality.

Like jasmine, the oil helps to reunite our emotional and sensual natures, aspects of being that need to contain each other and blend. If not, the Heart and Mind *(Shen)*, alienated from the tangible senses, easily become uprooted from the *yin*. Without the calm and stable residence of the moist *yin-energy*, restlessness and agitation may occur. Or emotions cannot flow and tend to "dry up", leading to isolation and depression. In either case, the Mind *(Shen)* loses its natural ability to express and experience both pleasure and joy.

Instilling us with the sweetness of peaceful paradise – yet revealing the spice of a tropical sun – ylang ylang oil both soothes and entices, opens and centres us. It allows us to inwardly unify and so outwardly merge.

RADHA AND KRISHNA
The love of the Hindu god Krishna for the milkmaid Radha symbolizes not only the union of the Masculine and Feminine but of spirit and matter. The image captures the ecstatic sense of merging that is inherent in ylang ylang oil.

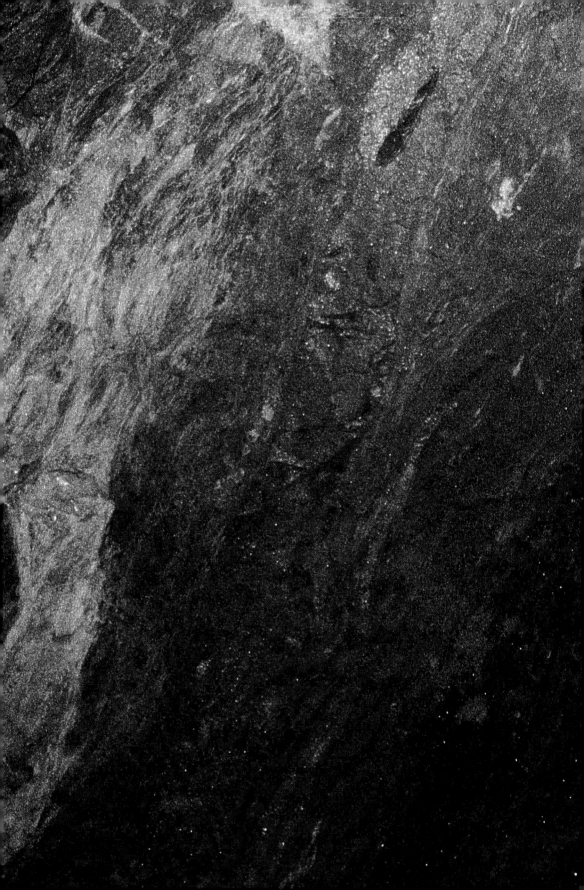

Part Three
Restoring Balance

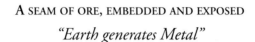

A SEAM OF ORE, EMBEDDED AND EXPOSED

"Earth generates Metal"

We have considered the mind and Spirit from the perspective of Oriental medicine, and have surveyed the energetics of 40 essential oils. In this third part, we apply this understanding to restoring emotional and mental balance. The psychological problems to receive our attention are those that are commonly encountered in daily life.

There are, of course, many ways that one can begin to restore balance – some ancient, others new. These include psychotherapy and counselling, meditation and yoga, relaxation exercises, spiritual healing and *tai ch'i*. Oriental medicine also places an emphasis on the importance of a healthy diet.

In order to obtain the best results from aromatherapy, it is often wise to combine the use of essential oils with one or more of these other methods. In addition, their effect will be optimized through applying them in two or three different ways – in the bath, burner or nebulizer, through aromatherapy massage, and through the application of aromatic creams to the wrists, temples, and neck.

You will find that stimulating the acupressure points illustrated in this part will enhance the effect of the oils still further. The treatment of the points may be incorporated into an entire aromatherapy massage sequence, or utilized on their own for a rapid-effect, "first aid" approach. Like the use of the oils, the acupressure points may be applied either in the treatment of others, or for purposes of self-treatment.

However, a number of the psychological complaints dealt with here are likely to require professional help, depending on the severity of the problem. One may need to consult a qualified psychotherapist or practitioner of traditional Oriental medicine.

All true healing takes time, and one should not expect results overnight – even when using the most appropriate oils. Although essential oils can have an immediate effect, most disharmonies of a protracted nature will take patience of Spirit to change.

Blending for Balance

the three levels of blending

There are various ways to approach the art of blending essential oils, depending upon the aim of the person selecting the oils. We can identify three overall *levels* of blending, each with its own specific goals. These are the *aesthetic*, the *clinical*, and the *psychological and spiritual.*

The blending of oils according to aesthetic principles is akin to the art of perfumery, and has as its aim the creation of a pleasing fragrance. You choose essences that *smell* nice together, based on their ability to harmonize with, and complement, each other.

To select oils that combine well on a sensory level, you should ideally "train" your nose, in order to discern the individual characteristics of a fragrance. When you can identify, within an essence, its principal aromatic qualities, you can then emphasize and modify their intensity through blending the oil with other essences. For example, the rich and tenacious aspects of rose oil will harmonize with those of patchouli, while blending rose with palmarosa oil will produce a more light and floral fragrance.

The clinical level of blending is concerned with the selection of oils for their *therapeutic* value. The aim here is to create a blend that will be of maximum benefit to the *health* of the individual. In traditional Chinese herbal medicine, individual remedies are selected to fill the therapeutic positions of Emperor, Minister, Assistant, and Messenger.

Let us take, as an example, the case of an individual with an asthmatic condition – one that involves mucus congestion and wheezing. Marjoram would make a very good Emperor oil, because of the all-round benefit it brings to the condition. Pine may be added as its Minister oil, to reinforce, in particular, the expectorant property of marjoram. As an Assistant oil, we could include that of clary sage, as it will assist and enhance the antispasmodic effect of the combination. Eucalyptus, finally, would make an effective Messenger oil, due to its capacity – among other properties – to direct the action of the blend toward the Lungs.

It is possible – even preferable – to incorporate within a

BLENDING FOR THE INDIVIDUAL
All essential oils have the power to affect us both emotionally and spiritually. Only those that are right for the individual – at that moment of their life – will possess the subtle potential to transform.

clinical approach to blending a degree of aesthetic criteria. That is, while still selecting oils for their therapeutic properties, we may emphasize those that blend well as fragrances.

The same may be applied to a psychological and spiritual approach to blending. This is blending at its most perceptive and discerning – one that places an emphasis on restoring emotional and mental balance. It is advisable, in this context, to restrict the number of oils in a blend to no more than three. The unique and subtle influence of each will only emerge if the blend is kept relatively simple. The following is an example.

A person suffers with feelings of restlessness and anxiety, brought on, in the main, by a particularly pressurized work situation. Due to apprehension about losing their job, they drive themselves to the point of exhaustion, yet cannot relax even when they try. There are also times when they become extremely tense and irritable, and very frustrated when something doesn't go to plan.

A disharmony within two of the Five Elements is present here. The individual's restlessness, anxiety, "driven" behaviour, and fear all indicate, at a fundamental level, an imbalance of the Will *(Zhi)* – pointing to distress within the Water Element. Their tension, irritability, and frustration reflect, in addition, stagnant *Qi-energy* and a problem with Wood. A combination of geranium and orange oils is called for, to pacify the Will and ease frustration.

While aesthetic blending relies on our "nose" – on our sensory discernment and flair – clinical blending depends upon our knowledge both of the oils and of common ailments. A psychological and spiritual approach, on the other hand, calls for a degree of "intuition" – of an ability to "sense" the condition of the Spirit. By "intuition", however, I do not refer to a *psychic* means of selection, but on a wisdom that comes through knowing the specific "character" of each essential oil, and of the states of mind that require their healing influence.

THE HARMONY OF THE FAMILY
As a general rule, the fragrances of essential oils that belong to the same plant family will tend to harmonize with, and enhance, each other. For example, orange, neroli, and bergamot oils – all members of the *Rutaceae* family – will blend very easily.

Nervous Tension & Agitation

oils that regulate and relax

Nervous tension is probably the most common psychological problem of all. Tension can, of course, be creative – and there are many who consider it an essential ingredient of their work and productivity. If, however, it becomes perturbing, draining, or difficult to contain, it clearly needs reducing.

There are many essential oils that, due to the intrinsically relaxing nature of their aroma and action, may be effectively used for both nervous tension and agitation. In contrast to tension, "agitation" is a more pronounced and acute form of mental-emotional disturbance – one that is characterized by extremely nervous and restless feelings.

Like all psychological problems, states of nervous tension are best approached with an eye to the individual concerned, taking into account the unique cause and characteristics of their particular disharmony. A blanket approach to the problem or problems will fail to yield the same results.

According to Oriental medicine, nervous tension and agitation are most frequently associated with the Heart and Liver, reflecting an imbalance within the Elements of Fire or Wood. Having said this, there are beneficial oils that can be more closely linked to the Earth, Water, and Metal Elements – and these should be remembered, too.

A tense state of mind and body represents, by its very nature, *stagnation of Qi* – that is, vital energy which has accumulated and become "stuck", inducing a taut, constricted feeling. The condition results from a failure of the Liver to perform its function of ensuring the smooth flow of *Qi-energy*. The oils of benefit have a *regulating* effect – by releasing and harmonizing "tensed up" vital energy, they diminish the pressure caused by emotional stress and mental strain.

The essential oils of Roman and German chamomile, sweet orange, and bergamot all work to relax nervous tension through regulating *Liver-Qi*. They are indicated, in particular, for the type of individual who becomes quickly aggravated by problems at work – or by situations that feel "out of control". Chamomile is suited to the kind of nervous

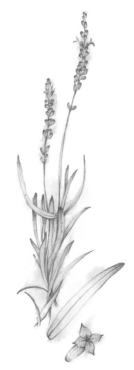

LAVENDER
The cool and soothing characteristic blue of lavender flowers relates to its ability to calm the mind and reduce inflammation. With the flowers perched on terminal spikes, high above grey-green clusters of leaves, they signify the capacity of the essential oil to lift us beyond the turmoil of anxiety and agitation.

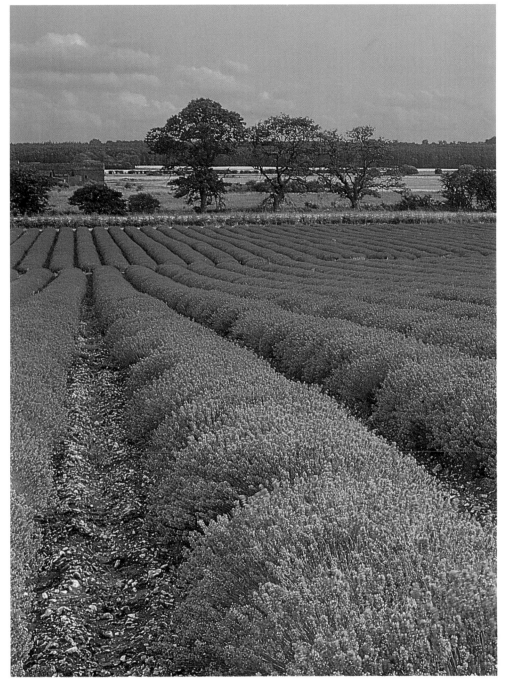

LAVENDER FIELDS

True lavender (Lavandula angustifolia) tends to flourish on the stony ground found at relatively high altitudes, well above the atmospheric haze that filters out a proportion of the sun's rays. Although it thrives in pure air, lavender produces more essential oil when grown on poor soil. It is an oil which restores calmness and clarity in the most unfavourable of circumstances.

tension that results from over-effort and over-control – typified by the perfectionist or "workaholic" person who is easily frustrated by obstacles. Bergamot oil, too, encourages us to "loosen up" and, like orange, can help to restore a sense of humour. Lavender and melissa oils also help to dissipate nervous tension. Not only do they smooth the flow of *Qi* and harmonize the Liver, but work in addition to calm the Heart and Mind *(Shen)*.

As the *Shen's* stable residence, the Heart is responsible for maintaining the overall balance of the psyche. All pressures of a mental-emotional nature will therefore have an energetic effect on the Heart. Most essential oils that are classified as *calmative* in nature – relaxing to the nervous system – subsequently help to harmonize the Heart and Mind *(Shen)*.

Lavender and melissa oils are indicated, in particular, for tension and agitation associated with *heat* in the Heart. *Heat* disturbs the Mind *(Shen)*, and produces a restless, sometimes hyperactive state that frequently results in insomnia.

Lavender and melissa oils are suited, emotionally, to the highly sensitive, sometimes introspective individual who finds it difficult to confront stressful situations. The oils not only benefit nervous tension but can help, in addition, to allay feelings of panic and hysteria.

Neroli, jasmine, and ylang ylang oils also calm the Heart – easing the tension of those who feel alienated from their senses and emotions. These are individuals who equate relaxation with directly relieving tension in the body.

As tonics of the *cool, moist yin-energy* of the Heart, rose and palmarosa oils calm tension and agitation when accompanied by thirst, dryness, night sweats, and insomnia. They are particularly relevant for the tension that results from emotional insecurity. Though its peaty scent does not appeal to all, spikenard is also indicated for agitated states of the Mind *(Shen)* – while the similarly "spiritual" oils of sandalwood and frankincense relax the nerves through calming the Intellect *(Yi)*. Frankincense, especially, may be used for the tension that has accumulated from excessive *mental* strain –

Suggested Blends
(no. of drops per 20ml/1tbsp of carrier)

AGGRAVATED & PRESSURIZED
chamomile (2), bergamot (2), orange (2)

NERVOUS & AGITATED
lavender (3), neroli (2), bergamot (1)

SUDDEN PSYCHOLOGICAL TRAUMA
lavender (3), frankincense (2), spikenard (1)

TENSE & EXHAUSTED
clary sage (3), cypress (2), lavender (1)

See Also

the type, for example, that results from exam revision.

Marjoram oil's sweet, herbaceous comfort appeals to those in whom there is a need to support the Earth Element. One may use it for states of nervous tension that swing between those of fatigue – the more tense one becomes, the more tired one gets. Clary sage oil possesses the same energetic property, and, like marjoram, is intrinsically "balancing". One of the most effective of antispasmodics, it works to eradicate tension through dispersing stagnant *Qi-energy*. Like cypress oil, it is indicated for premenstrual tension.

This brings us to geranium oil – like rose and palmarosa, a tonic of the *yin* energy. Its ability to settle and centre the Will *(Zhi)* makes it important for the kind of tension that drives one on – despite a feeling of exhaustion.

Acupressure treatment: Pericardium-6

Located on the front of the forearm, Pericardium-6 lies 2 cun (finger-widths) directly above the wrist crease, between the two tendons. Pericardium-6 smooths the flow of Qi in the Heart, and harmonizes and uplifts the Mind (Shen). Supporting the wrist with one hand, stimulate the pressure point by rubbing the thumb of the other hand in a circular motion over the point, with the fingers and palm of the hand clasping the back of the forearm. Stimulating Liver-3 will also benefit nervous tension.

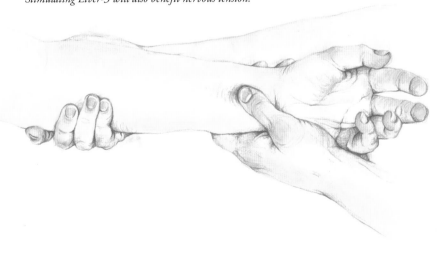

Overthinking & Worry

oils that settle the mind

In contrast to most other psychological problems, overthinking and worry relate to one main organ – the Spleen-pancreas. The residence of the Intellect *(Yi)*, the Spleen controls the thinking process, and lends to the Mind *(Shen)* the capacity for conceptualization.

When, due to worry, tension, or mental strain, the Intellect *(Yi)* is subjected to undue pressure, overthinking is likely to ensue. In this condition, thinking is hyperactive, and can become muddled, confused, and "bogged down". The Intellect *(Yi)* has difficulty in reaching clear conclusions, as the mind churns continually in an attempt to find them. Such a condition is an imbalance of Reflection – the root "emotion" of the Earth Element.

The essential oils that benefit overthinking, while they all help to harmonize the Earth Element, work to settle the mind in distinctly different ways. While some are grounding and comforting, others are regulating and clarifying – they can all play a role in addressing the problem.

The essential oils that are primarily grounding in influence are those of benzoin and vetiver. Sweet, resinous, and relaxing, they "earth" the *Qi* that has risen to the head, producing a mind full of superfluous thoughts. They are suited, in particular, to those who are physically inactive, and who have lost touch with the capacity to simply *be*.

Sandalwood, too, embodies the principle of *being* – an oil that lulls and deeply calms the mind. Draining conditions of congestion and *heat*, it quells the fixed and agitated thoughts that lead to mental obsessiveness. Its deeply soothing sweetness helps to replace a worried outlook with a more calmly reflective response to life's problems.

Frankincense and myrrh oils share with sandalwood an ability to instil tranquillity. Soothing and balsamic – on both physical and spiritual levels – frankincense eases the mind when troubled by thoughts of regret, and worries of a mundane kind. Just as lavender is indicated for the over-emotional type of person, frankincense oil is suited to those who are mentally overwhelmed.

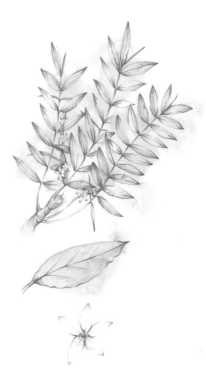

FRANKINCENSE
The oleo-gum-resin that forms in secreting canals within the phloem of the frankincense tree possesses the ability to transform from a liquid state to a solid one, following its contact with air. Frankincense oil is concerned with the transformation of the Self – from an amorphous state of spiritual consciousness into a crystallized one.

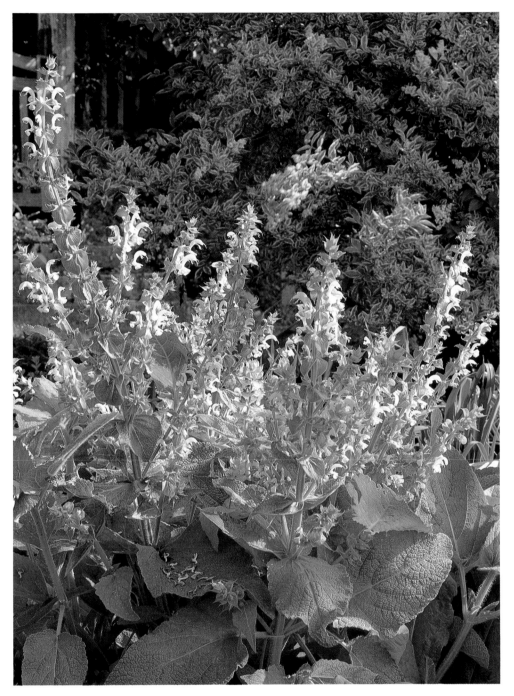

CLARY SAGE

For a plant with a non-woody stem, clary sage reaches a considerable
height, and has large, hairy, heart-shaped leaves that grow near the
ground. The contrast between these and its small, well-protected
flowers reminds us of the ability of the oil to reconcile extremes,
and so alleviate indecision.

The essential oils of marjoram and the chamomiles help to quell the worry of a mind under pressure and in need of comfort. Camphoraceous and clarifying, yet sweet and reassuring, marjoram oil is useful for hazy, fretful states of mental fatigue. It helps to settle those who feel they have no one to talk to, and must consequently struggle with their worries on their own. It is of benefit, in addition, for those whose tendency is to worry incessantly about others.

Roman and German chamomile oils are for the overthinking of the tense perfectionist, and for the person who finds it difficult to "switch off" from work.

Clary sage shares with the chamomile oils an ability to regulate and smooth the flow of *Qi*. It is recommended, in particular, for the type of overthinking that stems from a tense and changeable search for ideal solutions. Even when such a person has actually made a decision, they worry if it is right, and whether they should change their mind.

Fennel oil's ability to encourage self-expression benefits those whose tendency to worry is exacerbated by a difficulty with communication. Thoughts and concerns "ferment" because they have no positive outlet.

Patchouli oil, like vetiver, is rich and "grounding", restoring awareness of the body and senses. Earthy and sweet, it is supportive to the Spleen, and allays the worry that comes of excessive mental strain. Like coriander seed oil, patchouli gently stimulates the Mind *(Shen)*, and through its spicy warmth uplifts and arouses. Patchouli and coriander are suitable for the worry of the depressive, remote individual.

While clary sage and frankincense oils help to clarify and calm, those that excel in refreshing the mind are lemon and grapefruit oils. Lemon, in particular, clears mental "congestion" – the plethora of thoughts that "bog down" the mind. Though relatively mild in its action on the Intellect *(Yi)*, grapefruit, through its ability to regulate *Liver-Qi*, disperses the worry that stems from tension and frustration.

Geranium essential oil, like patchouli and vetiver, increases one's awareness of the senses. Sweet, floral, and astringent in

Suggested Blends
(no. of drops per 20ml /1tbsp of carrier)

OBSESSIVE OVERTHINKING
sandalwood (4), vetiver (2)

Over-PREOCCUPIED WITH DETAIL
frankincense (3), vetiver (2), lemon (1)

OVER-CONCERN FOR OTHERS
marjoram (3), chamomile (1), palmarosa (1)

OVER-ANALYTICAL & DETACHED
geranium (3), sandalwood (2) patchouli (1)

See Also

nature, it strengthens the energy of both the *yin* and the Spleen, and helps to settle a restless and scattered mind. It is indicated for those whose overthinking stifles and obscures the emotions. It may be used to encourage, in place of over-analysis, the capacity for receptivity and intuitive insight.

Cardamom oil combines a multiplicity of qualities, making it effective for worry in all its forms. Sweet, warm, and balsamic, it is by nature essentially "grounding" and comforting, and imbibes the Intellect *(Yi)* with contentment and tranquillity. It contains, at the same time, spicy, pungent notes that make it uplifting and clarifying. With such a synergy of psychological actions, cardamom conveys the *balanced* power of Earth – and benefits overthinking of the anxious, muddled, and depressive types.

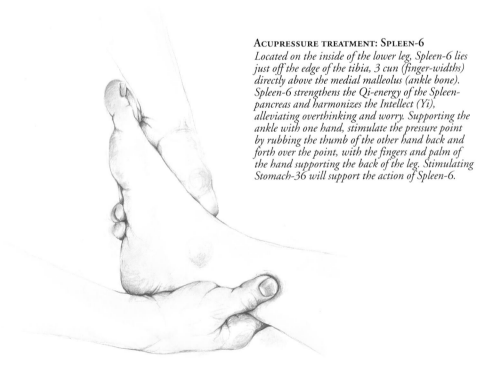

ACUPRESSURE TREATMENT: SPLEEN-6
Located on the inside of the lower leg, Spleen-6 lies just off the edge of the tibia, 3 cun (finger-widths) directly above the medial malleolus (ankle bone). Spleen-6 strengthens the Qi-energy of the Spleen-pancreas and harmonizes the Intellect (Yi), alleviating overthinking and worry. Supporting the ankle with one hand, stimulate the pressure point by rubbing the thumb of the other hand back and forth over the point, with the fingers and palm of the hand supporting the back of the leg. Stimulating Stomach-36 will support the action of Spleen-6.

Anxiety & Apprehension
oils that calm and reassure

According to Oriental medicine, the two organs that are most frequently in disharmony, in states of anxiety and apprehension are the Kidneys and the Heart.

The Kidneys are the residence of the Will *(Zhi)*. The source of our instinct for survival, they provide the psyche with the root emotion of Fear. Just as Anger, properly directed, is a positively assertive and creative force, so too does a potential capacity for Fear serve a necessary and deep-rooted purpose. Without it, we would lack our drive for self-preservation, and lose the wisdom gained from having a sense of our mortality.

When, due to instability of the Will *(Zhi)*, Fear becomes either inappropriate or excessive, it leads, however, to psychological disharmony. Fear can then express itself as a lack of self-confidence, a sense of apprehension, or a feeling of insecurity. These are signs of an imbalance within the Water Element. Among the oils that help to quell feelings of apprehension are those that reinforce the *Kidney-Qi* and the Will *(Zhi)*. These include thyme, juniper berry, and cypress.

Oil of thyme is best employed for fear of an *external* or *known* cause, and evokes the warrior that exists within us all. Juniper oil, too, is suitable for timidity and retreat, yet alleviates in addition an *inward* fear of failure. And while cedarwood oil may be employed for an inward fear of collapse, cypress oil is the choice for dread of a hidden or *unknown* origin.

States of anxiety are more commonly linked to an energetic imbalance of the Heart – the home of the Mind *(Shen)*. When the Heart is deficient in either *Qi*, *blood*, or *yin*, the Mind *(Shen)* becomes disturbed, and loses its settled state of residence. This results in feelings of emotional unease. Equally so, long-term emotional pressures that result in chronic anxiety can actually cause these energetic deficiencies, leading, in turn, to additional problems of a physiological nature. Anxiety, therefore, can be either a *cause* or a *symptom* of a disharmony of the Heart and Fire Element – in either case, the same oils will be of benefit.

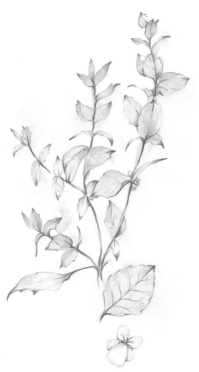

MELISSA
"Balm, cordial and exhilarating, sovereign for the brain, strengthening the memory, and powerfully chasing away melancholy. . . . The fresh sprigs gather'd, put into wine, or other drinks, during the heat of summer, give it a marvellous quickness." John Evelyn, 1699

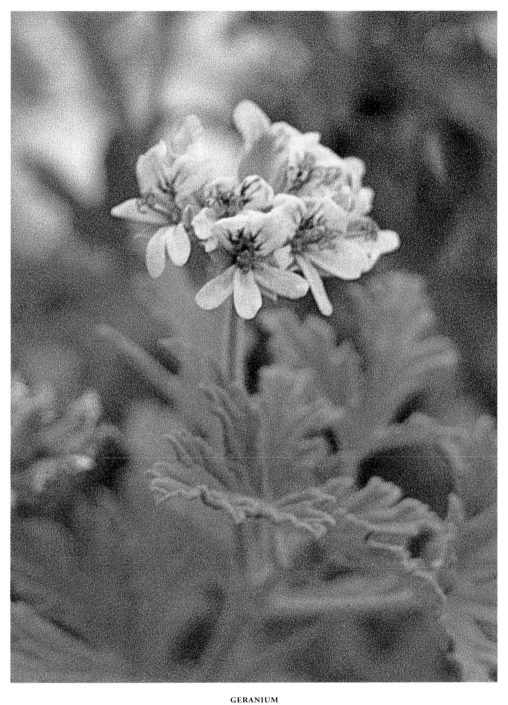

GERANIUM

*Although Geranium produces umbels of flowers, it is the hairy, lobed
leaves of the plant that yield the essential oil. It is unusual that the leaves
should be scented and not the flowers – and produce a fragrance that is
not just "green", but sufficiently floral to imitate rose.*

When the *cool*, sustaining *yin* of the Kidneys fails to nourish the *yin* of the Heart, anxiety, insecurity, night sweats, and insomnia can occur. The oils called for in this condition are geranium and vetiver. Geranium calms the nervous anxiety of those not by nature "emotional" – the "over-achievers" who have little time for feelings. Vetiver oil is similar in nature, helping to restore a sense of rooted stability to those who feel anxious and "disembodied". Both these oils may be used for fear and "panic attacks".

Rose and palmarosa oils, because they "nourish" the *Heart-yin*, have a cooling, calming, and supportive effect. Rose, in particular, is indicated for *deep* anxiety, and reassures those who, in emotional distress, cannot bear to be left alone. The oil alleviates anxiety that is caused by fear and insecurity – including a fear of "losing control". Like melissa, the slightly sour or astringent note in rose oil can help the Heart to "reabsorb" the Mind *(Shen)*.

Jasmine oil combines a calming effect with a distinctly uplifting one and is especially useful for anxiety when it alternates with feelings of depression. Ylang ylang oil is similar in nature – in both its aroma and energy – though it is better for "sedating" an extremely restless, racing mind.

Lavender and melissa oils both *cool* the Heart and smooth the flow of *Qi*, and are among the most comforting oils for the Mind *(Shen)*. While rose and palmarosa are for the abandoned and bereft, lavender and melissa are best employed for anxiety in those who feel oppressed and suffocated – by situations or other people. They are called for, in addition, for anxiety that is compounded by a sense of emotional confusion – where there is profound conflict of duties and desires, or the feeling of not knowing "where to turn".

Combined with cypress and neroli, lavender oil may be considered effective, in particular, for anxieties that are expressed through compulsive behaviour.

Neroli oil is of benefit for those who cannot confront painful and disturbing emotions – feelings of shame, guilt, or half-conscious hurt and rage. It helps, above all, to allevi-

Suggested Blends
(no. of drops per 20ml /1tbsp of carrier)

AGORAPHOBIA
juniper (2), cypress (2), true melissa (1)

SUDDEN FEAR, ESPECIALLY AT NIGHT
geranium (2), vetiver (2), rose (1)

ANXIOUS DESPERATION
lavender (3), rose (2)

HYPOCHONDRIA
lavender (3), cypress (3)

See Also

ate the anxiety of those who have despaired of finding peace of mind. Neroli not only calms and soothes the Mind *(Shen)* but restores a sense of hope to the Ethereal Soul *(Hun)*.

Like rose, jasmine, and ylang ylang, neroli oil, in addition, is suitable for sexual anxiety, and relieves the unease of those who feel ashamed of the body. Lavender oil, in contrast, is for those who are anxious for their health – or who have a tendency toward hypochondria. Spikenard oil, finally, may be used for "spiritual" anxiety – one that is characterized by a loss of faith. It settles and "earths" both the Mind *(Shen)* and Ethereal Soul *(Hun)*, and renews our trust in life when everything seems pitched against us. Combined with other anxiety-relieving oils, it will contribute a capacity for acceptance and transcendence.

ACUPRESSURE TREATMENT: HEART-7

Located on the front of the wrist, Heart-7 lies on the wrist crease, just inside the pisiform bone. It stabilizes the Qi of the Heart, and calms and comforts the Mind (Shen). Supporting the recipient's hand with one hand, stimulate the pressure point by rubbing the thumb of the other hand back and forth over the point, with the fingers and palm of the hand clasping the back of the wrist. Stimulating Kidney-6 will also help to alleviate anxiety and apprehension.

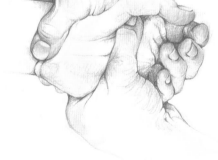

Poor Concentration & Memory

oils that clarify the mind

There are, in terms of traditional Oriental medicine, a number of factors that influence the power of concentration and memory. The condition of the *blood,* the Heart and circulation, and of the Spleen-pancreas and Kidneys are all an influence on the strength of the conscious mind. Consequently, there are a number of essential oils that improve the ability to concentrate and remember, depending upon the nature of the disharmony involved.

Rosemary oil is one of the most fundamental and well known of these. Its ability to promote the arterial circulation of blood, together with its action to move *Qi* upward, makes it one of the most powerful of *cephalic* essential oils – those that stimulate cerebral activity. In its ability to promote both concentration and presence of mind, it is rivalled only by essential oil of basil *(Ocinum basilicum).* Regrettably, however, even the oil of European or French basil *(Ocinum basilicum var. album)* can contain sufficient amounts of methyl chavicol (estragole) to throw into doubt the complete safety of its use.

Like rosemary, laurel oil strengthens the *Qi* of the Heart and enhances one's presence of mind. While rosemary may be utilized for poor concentration generally – especially when there is nervous debility – the use of laurel oil is best reserved for those engaged in study and learning.

Tea tree is both a cardiac and nervous tonic, and like rosemary invigorates the cerebral flow of blood. It is suitable primarily for those whose concentration has been adversely affected by poor vitality and health.

Rosemary, laurel, and tea tree oils are not only called for in states of mental fatigue but can also improve poor memory. An age-old Herb of Remembrance, rosemary, in particular, is renowned for this ability. As a tonic of the Heart, it is considered, according to Oriental medicine, to prevent the loss of *long-term* memory.

Turning our attention from the Fire to the Earth Element, we should consider next the important role of the Spleen. The residence of the Intellect *(Yi),* the Spleen-pancreas is

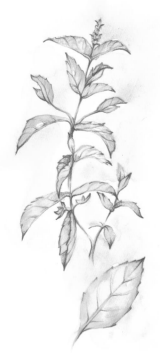

PEPPERMINT
"Touching garden Mint, as the very smell of it alone recovereth and refresheth the spirits, so the taste stirreth up the appetite . . . . The juice of Mints is excellent for to scoure the pipes and clear the voice, being drunk a little before a man is to strain himself either in the choir, or upon the stage, or at the bar."
Pliny, AD 77 (translated by Holland, 1601)

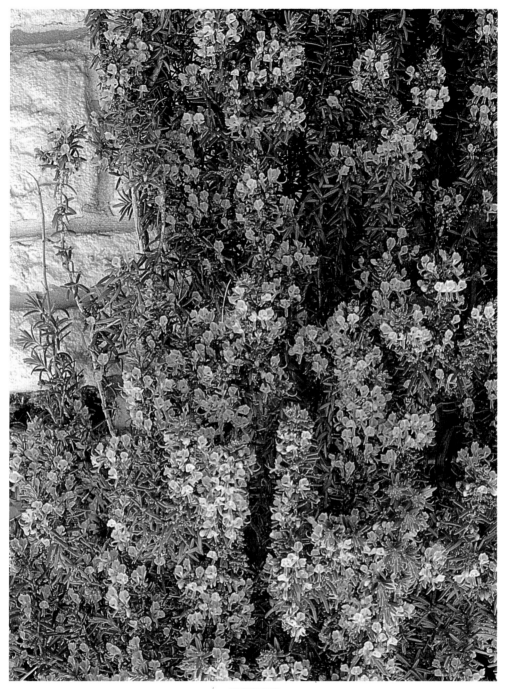

ROSEMARY

*"As for Rosmarine, I let it run all over my garden walls, not only because
my bees love it, but because it is the herb sacred to remembrance,
and, therefore, to friendship; whence a sprig of it hath a dumb
language that maketh it the chosen emblem of our funeral wakes
and in our burial grounds."*
Sir Thomas More, 16th century

responsible for thinking, concentration, logic, and analysis. Just as it controls, with the help of the Stomach, the digestion and transformation of food, so does it govern the digestion of information – the absorption and analysis of mental stimuli.

Two of the best essential oils to strengthen the mental function of the Spleen are cardamom and coriander seed. Not only are they useful as digestive stimulants but are classified, in addition, as neurotonic oils. Cardamom oil enhances our curiosity and retentiveness, while coriander seed invigorates the mind's creativity.

Marjoram, as well, is a traditional cephalic, and was used by Dioscorides to warm and buttress the nerves. Like clary sage oil, it improves the concentration of those who are both tired and tense.

Clary sage itself is renowned for promoting clarity, and shares with common sage *(Salvia officinalis)* an ability to strengthen the power of judgment. Its traditional reputation as a Visionary Herb reflects its potential to stimulate "higher" thought, and aid the Intellect *(Yi)* in its intuitive function. It is in this way similar to frankincense oil, the ancient aromatic of contemplation. Frankincense oil relaxes and, at the same time, rejuvenates the mind, expanding awareness and uplifting the Spirit. It may be used to initiate a tranquil type of concentration, and to cultivate a meditative, single-pointed focus. It can also be helpful for staying mentally calm and clear, and is the oil to sniff in exams!

One of the most clarifying oils for the Intellect *(Yi)* is lemon. Light and refreshing in nature, it is indicated for the heavy-headed and congested individual whose concentration is "muzzy" and dull. It helps, in addition, to maximize learning and memory – especially of details and numerous facts.

Perhaps the most effective stimulant of the learning process is peppermint oil. While the oils so far analysed have related to the Heart and Spleen, the action of peppermint pertains more to the Stomach, and promotes, in particular, the ability to "absorb". A nervous stimulant that amplifies

Suggested Blends

(no. of drops per 20ml/1tbsp of carrier)

AS A STUDY AID
rosemary (4), laurel (1), peppermint (1)

VAGUE & INDECISIVE
clary sage (3), rosemary (2)

RESTLESS & DISTRACTED
frankincense (3), geranium (2)

FORGETFUL
pine (3), lemon (1), rosemary (1)

See Also

Cardamom *pp.56-7*
Clary sage *pp.62-3*
Coriander *pp.64-5*
Frankincense *pp.74-5*
Geranium *pp.76-7*
Hyssop *pp.82-3*
Laurel *pp.88-9*
Lemon *pp.92-3*
Marjoram *pp.94-5*
Peppermint *pp.108-9*
Pine *pp.110-11*
Rosemary *pp.114-15*
Tea tree *pp.120-1*
Thyme *pp.122-3*

the Intellect, it helps us to listen, to take in, and digest.

Hyssop, thyme, and pine essential oils improve concentration through warming and tonifying the *yang*. Each possessing a neurotonic potential, they are useful to invigorate the mind in conditions of nervous exhaustion.

Because they tonify the *Kidney-Qi*, thyme and pine oils are, in addition, indicated for loss of *short-term* memory. Combined with rosemary oil, they may be used to good effect for poor memory in the elderly, where a decline in genetic essence has led to cerebral insufficiency. If the constitution of such a person is *hot, dry,* and restless, then a tonic of the Kidneys' *yin-energy* is required. Geranium essential oil may therefore be used in their place.

ACUPRESSURE TREATMENT: GALL BLADDER-20
Located on the back of the neck, just below the base of the skull, Gall Bladder-20 lies in the hollow behind the bony prominence behind the ear. It clears the mind, improves concentration and strengthens memory. Supporting the forehead with one hand, stimulate the pressure point by rubbing the thumb of the other hand in a circular motion over the point. Stimulating Small Intestine-3 will support the action of Gall Bladder-20.

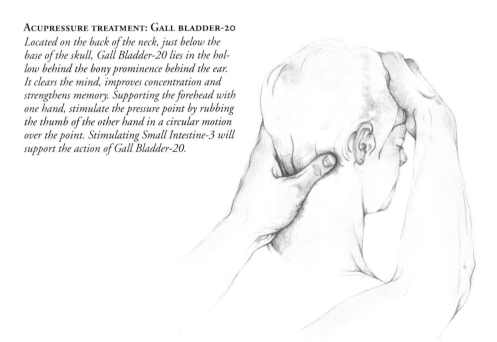

Lack of Confidence & Self-Esteem

oils that boost morale

Through housing the Mind *(Shen)* – the focus of the Self – the Heart is the organ most responsible for maintaining a sense of confidence and morale. The central organ of the Fire Element, it dominates self-expression, presence of mind, and overall emotional harmony.

It is supported in this role by the Kidneys, home of the Will *(Zhi)*. The Will roots the Mind *(Shen)* and provides it with determination and with an instinctive feeling of self-assurance, of belief in our innate capacities. The main organ of the Water Element, the Kidneys in disharmony produce fear and timidity, and weaken resolve in difficult situations.

Finally, the Lungs contribute to a sense of self-confidence by maintaining our psychological "boundary". If this becomes blurred, we feel exposed and vulnerable, preferring to withdraw and to avoid the risk of contact. In keeping with the Metal Element, the Lungs in harmony provide verve and optimism, and are, in addition, a source of self-respect.

One of the most effective aromatics for boosting self-confidence is rosemary oil. A tonic of the *Heart-, Lung-* and *Kidney-Qi*, it warms and invigorates both the body and mind, uplifting the Spirit and instilling inspiration. The focus of rosemary's subtle psychological action is on the Mind *(Shen)* and the Fire Element. Here, its ability to reinforce self-identity makes it applicable for both a lack of purpose and self-esteem.

An age-old emblem of noble accomplishment, laurel is also indicated for low self-esteem – the type that results from poor intellectual and artistic confidence. Its influence, again, centres on the Heart and Fire Element, inspiring within the Mind *(Shen)* a spirit of creative boldness.

Jasmine oil, too, encourages creativity, uplifting the Mind *(Shen)* in a gentle and sensuous way. Warm and reassuring in its fragrance and effect, it helps to free us from unnecessary self-restraint, relaxing the mind and harmonizing the Heart. Jasmine oil enhances the confidence that comes from being consistently true to oneself. Rose oil works in a similar way to jasmine, comforting the Mind *(Shen)* in states of emotion-

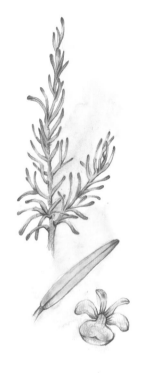

ROSEMARY
Everything about rosemary is ascending – its tall, erect stem, its long, slender branches, and its upright leaves. Even the pungent nobility of its strong, fresh scent lifts our spirits skyward, while the vital action of the essence raises the Qi and blood to brain.

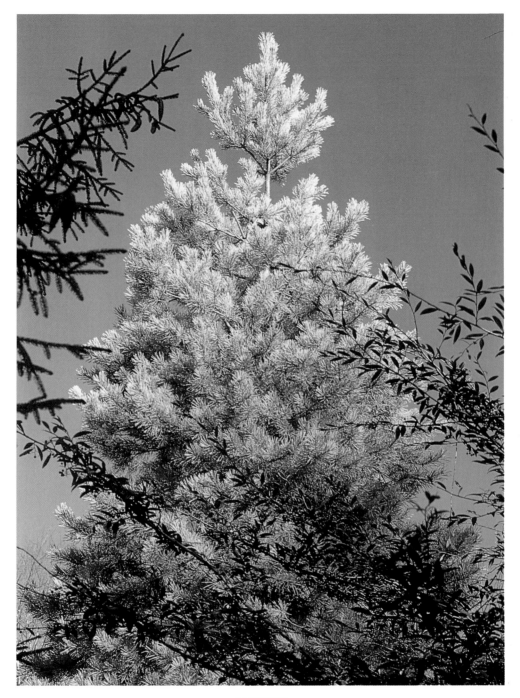

SCOTS PINE

Pinus sylvestris – "the pine of the woods" – favours the alpine mountainsides of northern zones, and braves scanty sunlight and freezing temperatures. Like the eternal Tree of Life, it concentrates within itself an inner light and warmth, and conveys the exhilarating freshness of its environment through the fragrance of its needles.

al alienation. It is recommended for a loss of self-esteem of the very deepest kind – where emotional pain has injured the capacity for self-love.

The role of fennel oil is a supportive one – of benefit to those whose lack of self-assurance stems from an inability to fully express themselves. Oil of ginger, on the other hand, can boost the confidence of those who lack initiative. Not only does it rouse the Will *(Zhi)* of the Kidneys, but through its spicy, invigorating warmth can restore the morale of the Mind *(Shen)*.

Perhaps the most potent essential oil for low morale is that of common thyme. A deeply fortifying neurotonic, it was considered by tradition to both dispel melancholy and promote bravery. Its ability to empower the Will and "open the chest" helps us to overcome feelings of self-doubt and defeatism. A more energetically *cool* and gentle alternative to common thyme *(Thymus vulgaris thymoliferum)* is that of geranium-scented thyme *(Thymus vulgaris geranioliferum)*, an oil with similar psychological benefits.

While rosemary and laurel are represented astrologically by the Sun – symbol of the individual – thyme and juniper berry are associated with Mars, an emblem of assertiveness and fiery self-assurance.

Like oil of common thyme, juniper berry augments the Will of the Kidneys and helps to free us from states of psychological "contraction". It benefits individuals who, burdened and withdrawn, have lost their sense of *social* self-confidence – as well as their basic resilience and optimism.

Pine and hyssop oils should also be considered here – restoring confidence through their effect on the Bodily Soul *(P'o)*. Like oil of thyme, they "open the chest" and revive the spirits, dispelling the gloom of a negative outlook. Traditional Herbs of Protection, pine and hyssop are indicated for the person who is easily affected by an oppressive environment.

They share, with yarrow essential oil, an ability to reinforce the Metal Element, helping to counteract a feeling of vulner-

Suggested Blends
(no. of drops per 20ml / 1tbsp of carrier)

POOR INTELLECTUAL
SELF-CONFIDENCE
rosemary (3), laurel (2)

LACK OF SELF-WORTH
rose (2), jasmine (2)

LOW MORALE
thyme (2), pine (2), cedarwood (2)

WITHDRAWN & DEFEATIST
juniper (2), thyme (2)

See Also

Caraway pp.54-5
Cedarwood pp.58-9
Fennel pp.72-3
Ginger pp.78-9
Hyssop pp.82-3
Jasmine pp.84-5
Juniper pp.86-7
Laurel pp.88-9
Pine pp 110-11
Rose pp 112-13
Rosemary pp.114-15
Tea tree pp 120-1
Thyme pp.122-3
Yarrow pp.126-7

ability. Yarrow can help to restore those whose self-esteem has been wounded by both psychological and physical abuse.

The psychological action of tea tree oil also relates to Metal – a major tonic of the Lungs and *Defensive-Qi.* With a concomitant action on the *yang* of the Heart, it is indicated primarily for the despondency and loss of confidence that arises through struggles with one's health.

While tea tree bolsters our endurance in poor health, cedarwood oil helps to promote psychological stamina generally. Tonifying the *Kidney-Qi* and fortifying the Will *(Zhi),* it sustains our confidence and morale in hardship of every kind. Caraway oil, on the other hand, strengthens our confidence to make and keep commitments. It deepens our sense of resolve when we feel like "giving up".

Acupressure treatment: Kidney-3

Located on the inside of the ankle, Kidney-3 lies halfway between the medial malleolus (ankle bone) and the posterior edge of the Achilles tendon. Kidney-3 supports the Qi of the Kidneys and reinforces the Will (Zhi), helping to restore confidence and courage. Supporting the heel with one hand, stimulate the pressure point by rubbing the thumb of the other hand up and down over the point. Stimulation of Heart-5 uplifts the Mind (Shen), and will help to counteract poor self-esteem.

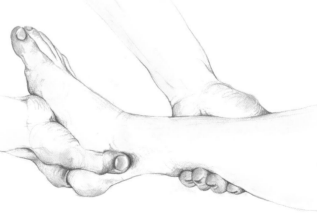

Anger & Frustration
oils that pacify the spirit

Most of the essential oils that relieve frustration, irritability, and resentment have an energetic effect on the Liver. According to Oriental medicine, the root emotion of the Liver, and of the Wood Element generally, is that of Anger. Although anger is generally considered to be a negative feeling, it is viewed from the Oriental perspective as encapsulating a necessary, and potentially creative, force. It is an extension, energetically, of the Liver's capacity for assertiveness. It is only viewed as "negative" when out of balance or control – when Anger is excessive or "deficient".

An excessive accumulation of Anger, like a feeling of frustration, is invariably a sign of stagnation of *Qi* – whether or not the reasons for such feelings are adequate or justified. The aim of "treatment" through aromatherapy can either be to pacify anger that is inappropriate, or to relieve the tension of those whose irritation is understandable. As with the treatment of any psychological disharmony, the helper/therapist should naturally remain wholeheartedly non-judgmental.

The ultimate aim of pacifying anger is to restore to the Ethereal Soul *(Hun)* – the spirit housed by the Liver – its innate capacity for tolerance and human kindness.

We can begin by considering the action of three citrus essential oils – orange, bergamot, and grapefruit – each of which helps to regulate the Liver and smooth the flow of *Qi*. Oil of sweet orange, with its warm, sunny, and fruity aroma, is excellent for tense, frustrated states – especially in those who anticipate obstacles. It is ideal for those who "fly into a rage" when mechanical objects won't function properly. The effect of bergamot oil is very similar, and helps to defuse an angry attitude through encouraging a spirit of compromise.

Grapefruit oil is not as relaxing as those of orange and bergamot, yet is particularly cleansing and refreshing. It is indicated, especially, for *repressed* or *sustained* feelings of anger – those which have developed into smouldering resentment, or are expressed through over-eating.

Peppermint oil, too, may be used for frustrated overeating, but it is indicated mainly for a lack of tolerance. Freeing

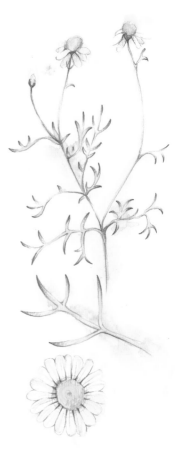

CHAMOMILE
"The Chamomile shall teach thee patience
That rises best when trodden upon."
Old English saying

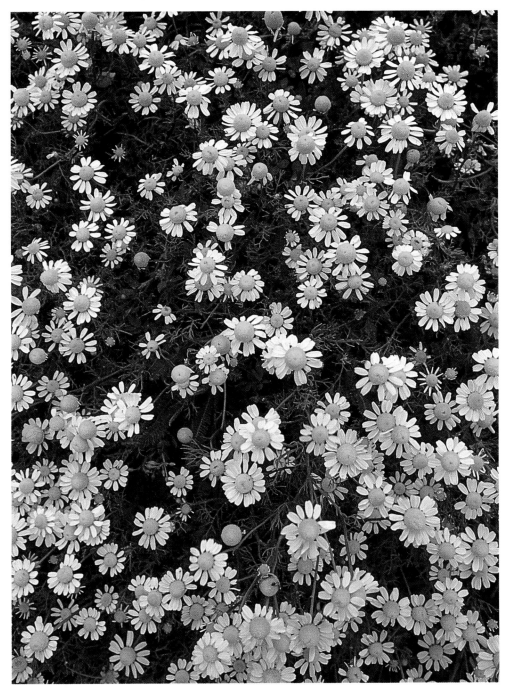

CHAMOMILE FLOWERS

The open-hearted innocence of the daisy-like flowers of German chamomile remind us of the oil's ability to restore tolerance and contentment. The fact that they are composite – each flowering head composed of numerous, tiny florets – suggests, in addition, the power to unify and harmonize.

constraint in the flow of *Liver-Qi* and enhancing the ability to "absorb", it helps to "swallow" what we may find difficult, and to "let go" of stubbornness and fixed resistance.

Another group of beneficial essential oils are provided by the *Compositae* family. Roman and German chamomile, yarrow, and everlasting work to both smooth the *Liver-Qi* and clear *Liver-heat,* and help to pacify an angry Spirit.

The chamomiles are, to my mind, the two most important essential oils for problems of anger, and help to soothe feelings of resentment in almost any circumstance. They are suited, in particular, for the type of individual who becomes angry because they feel neglected – even though they deny that they need or expect support. Theirs is often the kind of anger that we could also describe as "moody" – a sullen irritability that frequently comes and goes.

Yarrow oil may prove to be of benefit for similar states of mind – ideally suited to the anger of the individual who is easily threatened and defensive, ready to take offence at the slightest hint of criticism. Yarrow is also indicated, however, for the anger that lies buried beneath a deep sense of wounding – the Spirit stricken by unexpressed rage. The resulting dejection and despair can only disperse when the person in question begins to "own" their anger.

Oil of everlasting is also appropriate for the repressed type of anger – particularly when it has developed into long-standing resentment. It works to dissolve the bitterness of the person who continually bears a grudge, helping to restore a capacity for forgiveness and compassion.

Let us now turn to lavender oil – beneficial for tension and frustration generally. Calming the Heart as well as smoothing the flow of *Qi,* lavender is one of the most effective oils for pent-up feelings of annoyance. It may be used, in addition, to relax the nerves after sudden outbursts of rage.

Oil of rose is best reserved for the anger of those who feel hurt. It is recommended, in particular, for the resentment that results from emotional coldness, rejection, and betrayal. Clearing *heat* from both the Liver and Heart, it is useful, in

Suggested Blends
(no. of drops per 20ml/1tbsp of carrier)

FRUSTRATED & IRRITABLE
orange (2), bergamot (2), chamomile (2)

IMPATIENT & INTOLERANT
bergamot (3), lavender (2), peppermint (1)

TOUCHY & DEFENSIVE
yarrow (4), chamomile (1)

HURT & BITTER
rose (2), lavender (2), everlasting (1)

See Also
Bergamot pp.52-3
Chamomile pp.60-1
Everlasting pp.70-1
Grapefruit pp.80-1
Lavender pp.90-1
Orange pp.102-3
Rose pp.112-13
Spikenard pp.118-19
Yarrow pp.126-7

addition, for those who become angry and later regret it, and are filled with painful remorse.

Like everlasting, the action of spikenard oil reaches far into the psyche, and works to soften the Ethereal Soul *(Hun)* when we are hardened with immovable hostility. Although the healing process involved may be a slow one, spikenard is appropriate for a deep bitterness of Spirit – where resentment has blocked both spiritual growth and happiness.

ACUPRESSURE TREATMENT: GALL-BLADDER-34

On the outside of the upper leg, Gall Bladder-34 lies in the hollow slightly below and in front of the head of the fibula bone. Gall Bladder smooths the flow of Liver-Qi, eases nervous and muscular tension, and harmonizes the Ethereal Soul (Hun). Supporting the leg with one hand, stimulate the pressure point by rubbing the thumb of the other hand in a circular motion over the point. Stimulation of Liver-3 will also help to relieve frustration, irritability, and resentment.

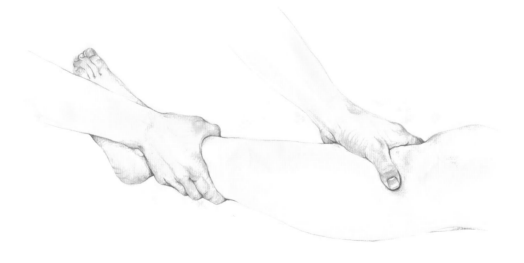

Disempowerment & Indecision
oils that fortify the Spirit

The essential oils that benefit conditions of disempowerment are those that promote will-power, fortify endurance, and enhance vitality of spirit. Like the oils that are indicated for poor confidence and apprehension, they tend on the whole to tonify the *yang* energy of the body/mind – and are energetically *warm* as a result.

In terms of the Five Elements, we may consider first the oils that strengthen the Water Element – such as essential oil of ginger. Ginger empowers our ability to take swift and affirmative action, warming the *yang* of the Kidneys and augmenting the Will *(Zhi)*. Its parallel effect on the Heart and Mind *(Shen)* makes it an ideal oil for apathy.

The effect of juniper berry oil is similar, if wider. Suited to those who tend to isolate themselves in difficulty, it drives away doubts and breaks through defeatism, restoring our resolve to surmount life's obstacles. Cedarwood oil, in contrast, holds us steady and firm, and fortifies the Will *(Zhi)* through reinforcing stamina. With the potential to impart a sense of spiritual resilience, it enables us to transform a victimized attitude into one of imperturbable strength.

Thyme essential oil empowers in a number of ways. Not only does it help to boost confidence and morale but will, in addition, benefit those who have difficulty being assertive, and who, allowing others to "dominate the agenda", later regret their compliance.

Like thyme essential oil, hyssop and pine oils revitalize the Bodily Soul *(P'o)*, and strengthen the function of the Defensive-Qi. They are recommended, in this respect, for the vulnerability and escapism that results from a weakness of the Metal Element, and from a lack of vital force. They empower us to participate fully in the world, and yet to maintain distinction and boundary. Hyssop and pine oils are helpful, therefore, for those who are particularly sensitive to a negative, "draining" environment, and who are easily exhausted by a stressful atmosphere.

Eucalyptus oil, too, has a pungent, "opening" effect, empowering those who feel trapped and "suffocated".

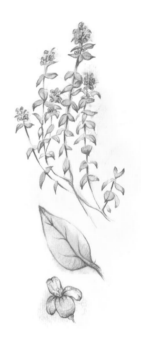

THYME
"Thyme is good against the Sciatica, the pain in the side and breast, against the wind in the side and belly, and is profitable also for such as are fearful, melancholic, and troubled in mind."
John Gerard, 1597

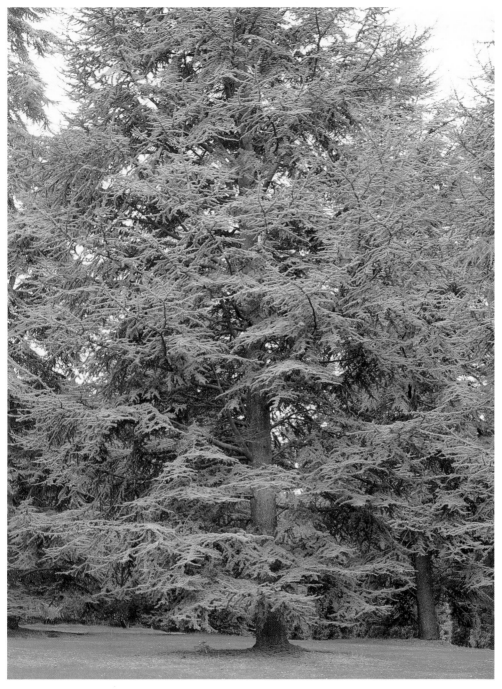

CEDAR TREE

*The majestic shape of cedar, sturdy and serene, beckons those in
need of reassurance to stand before its towering fortitude, just as one
would before a wise, compassionate elder. The essence that it offers us
possesses a deep and ancient strength.*

Instilling a sense of freedom, it invigorates the Spirit, and inspires an urge for a wider experience of life.

All the essential oils associated with the Metal Element enhance our ability to relinquish the outworn. Their generally fresh and clarifying nature encourages us to be fully present in the moment, ready to embrace each new experience. There is no essential oil better to demonstrate this power than that of cypress.

Dispersing stagnation in both the Bodily Soul *(P'o)* and Will *(Zhi)*, cypress oil allows us to let go of the past, and to initiate or accept changes now necessary or unavoidable. Suitable, in particular, for loss and disappointment – as well as compulsiveness and fear – it enhances our ability to transform and renew. Cypress, in addition, helps to bring to the surface difficult emotions that have been repressed – especially those that disempower the psyche through finding expression in self-destructive ways.

Benzoin oil, too, is helpful in times of change – though in a different way to cypress. Warm and stabilizing, it reassures and strengthens, alleviating worry and nervous fatigue. Caraway, in contrast, affords the power of stamina, helping us to adhere to chosen goals. Though the context of their use may differ, both benzoin and caraway promote inner stability, and through the power of Earth work to steady our course.

Clary sage oil couples the realism of the Earth Element with the vibrant force of Metal. It promotes insight, decisiveness, and a lucid and instinctive certainty. It can be used for tense and fatigued individuals who, due to a sense of confusion and distraction, fail to find the answers to their problems. Feeling "lost" and "in a haze", they find it difficult to take a clear and decisive course of action.

Other essential oils of benefit for indecision include those that regulate the *Liver-* and *Gall Bladder-Qi*. The Liver, according to Oriental medicine, is considered the "planner" of the body/mind – while the Gall Bladder (its paired organ) is the "decision-maker". When the organs of the Wood Element suffer with stagnant *Qi-energy*, disorganization and

Suggested Blends
(no. of drops per 20ml/1tbsp of carrier)

LACK OF DETERMINATION
cedarwood (4), ginger (2)

VULNERABLE & UNASSERTIVE
pine (3), thyme (2)

RESISTANT TO CHANGE
cypress (3), juniper (2), benzoin (1)

CHRONIC INDECISIVENESS
clary sage (3), bergamot (2), orange (1)

See Also

indecision arise. In this instance, the citrus oils may be used – bergamot, orange, and grapefruit, in particular. Just as they alleviate spasm on an energetic, physiological level, so, too, do they regulate the "spasmodic" behaviour that results from continual changes of mind.

The ability of rosemary to strengthen one's sense of self makes it another particularly empowering aromatic. Energizing the Will *(Zhi)* and uplifting the Mind *(Shen)*, it encourages self-confidence and belief in one's destiny. Its parallel action on the Liver and Ethereal Soul *(Hun)* – one of strong invigoration – also helps us to set clear and attainable goals, and to resist being swayed by undue influences.

ACUPRESSURE TREATMENT: SMALL INTESTINE-3
Located on the outside of the hand, Small Intestine-3 lies immediately below the metacarpo-phalangeal joint of the little finger. Small Intestine-3 clarifies the mind, strengthens the Will (Zhi) and reinforces the ability to make decisions. Supporting the recipient's hand with one hand, stimulate the pressure point by rubbing the thumb of the other hand back and forth over the point. Stimulation of Kidney-3 will also benefit feelings of disempowerment.

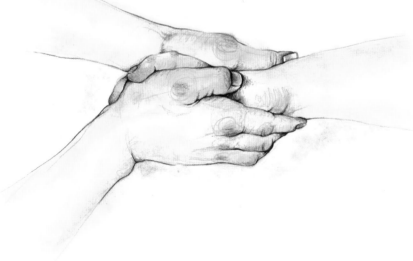

Depression & Negativity
oils that uplift the Spirit

There is a wide range of psychological issues and pressures that can lead to feelings of depression and negativity. The exact nature of the depression may be identified, through its emotional cause and characteristics, with one of the Five Elements. The Element to which the problem is linked is the one that we can most clearly associate with the precise feelings involved. In cases where we can perceive a disharmony of, say, two Elements, we may combine two or three essential oils that address the emotional issues connected with each. There are, in addition, a number of oils that unquestionably work on more than just one Element, and these will be particularly useful in such instances.

Depression of a Wood Nature

Because it ensures the smooth flow of *Qi-energy*, the Liver seeks to bestow an easy-going, carefree attitude. The harmonious movement of *Qi* is crucial for maintaining our overall emotional wellbeing, as feelings must ebb and *flow*. When, due to mounting pressures, tension takes hold, the *Qi* can stagnate and frustrate the Spirit, leading to a sense of oppression. This is a pattern that makes itself evident through the depression that follows long-term stress. It is most commonly seen in hard-working, ambitious individuals who suddenly lose motivation and drive. Either the self-imposed pressure becomes too great and they suddenly "collapse" within, or they are forced to give up cherished employment, depriving their lives of meaning. In both cases, their depression involves loss of purpose and "vision".

Resolute purpose and vision is a central faculty of the Ethereal Soul *(Hun)*. When chronic tension, frustration, and resentment impede its free and easy movement, the Ethereal Soul loses its ability to motivate, seek, and aspire. While in harmony, it affords the capacity for hope, it now becomes a source of despair.

Bergamot oil has a wide reputation for a capacity to gently uplift – a direct result of its action of smoothing the flow of *Liver-Qi*. Combining an ability to both relax the nerves and

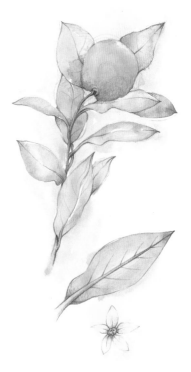

BERGAMOT
"Bergamot oil is the most bitter of all oils derived from Bitter oranges. In this respect Bergamot has an especially pronounced stimulating effect on the Liver, Stomach and Spleen; gastric stagnation due to weakness and deficiency is mobilised, and not only is the heaviness and distention relieved, but also the despondency and gloom which usually attend this type of condition are banished."
Peter Holmes, *The Energetics of Western Herbs*

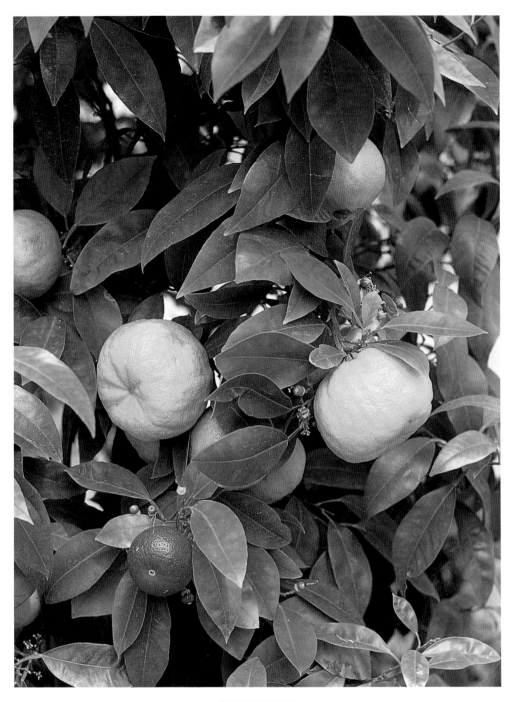

SWEET ORANGES

*The sweetness and succulence of the fruit of the orange tree make it, in
China, an emblem of good fortune. The fact that orange is a colour that is
considered to symbolize joy no doubt contributes to this view. Certainly,
the essence of the fruit, like the warmth of the sun, conveys a feeling of
happiness and wellbeing.*

refresh the Spirit, it is suitable for depressive states that stem from stress and pent-up feelings. The oils of sweet orange and mandarin *(Citrus reticulata)* work in a similar way, regulating the *Liver-Qi* and so easing depressive stress. Their warm, fresh, and fruity aromas are inherently joyful and harmonizing, particularly where tension has bred a narrow, negative outlook. Both evoke the carefree playfulness of the positive "inner child".

Neroli oil, like orange, regulates the *Qi* and, like jasmine oil, comforts the Mind *(Shen)*. It is called for, at a primary level, for the type of depression that comes of nervous and emotional exhaustion. It is indicated, at a more subtle level, for the despair of individuals who have cut themselves off from their senses and feelings, in order to escape emotional pain. Neroli uplifts the Spirit through its potential to nourish and unify. It can help to retrieve the repressed emotions which, until they are liberated, so often result in depression. Feelings of grief, abandonment, shame, and anger, stored in the musculature, may surface to consciousness, freeing the soul from their injury.

German and Roman chamomile oils are best employed for the moody, irritable type of depression associated, again, with stagnant *Liver-Qi*. Individuals prone to this condition are frequently dissatisfied with life, becoming frustrated with others and themselves. Symbolic of "patience in adversity", chamomile comforts the pain of the thwarted ego and helps to free the Spirit from its oppressive tyranny. Everlasting oil, too, can have a liberating effect – untying the depressive "knot" formed through emotional repression. It is helpful for those in whom anger has turned inward to engender a deep bitterness of Spirit, undermining hope and trust. Everlasting oil works to restore to the Ethereal Soul *(Hun)* its true compassion and vision, and alleviates depressive brooding.

Another member of the *Compositae* family is yarrow, used by the Orkney islanders for melancholy. It is applicable for those in whom negativity and depression spring from a sense of victimization. The hurt they carry has never really healed,

Suggested Blends
(no. of drops per 20ml/1tbsp of carrier)

FRUSTRATED, TENSE, & NEGATIVE
bergamot (3), orange (2), neroli (1)

BITTER & BROODING
chamomile (2), bergamot (2) everlasting (2)

SULLEN & WOUNDED
yarrow (4), hyssop (2)

SELF-CONDEMNATION
spikenard (2), lavender (2), rose (1)

See Also
Bergamot pp.52-3
Chamomile pp.60-1
Everlasting pp.70-1
Neroli pp.100-1
Orange pp.102-3
Spikenard pp.118-19
Yarrow pp.126-7

and cannot be given expression. They fear that by doing so, the pain would never cease to flow.

What the oils for depression of a Wood nature have in common is the potential to help release from the Ethereal Soul *(Hun)* a sense of obstruction and discontentment. Only then can one hope to restore to the Spirit the power of forgiveness and compassion.

There is no one for whom we need a more generous attitude than for ourselves. When, due to deep frustration and resentment, the Ethereal Soul becomes embittered and negative, we lose the tolerance not just for others but for ourselves – especially for our "faults" and limitations.

Spikenard oil may be used for the type of depression that results from an intolerance of oneself. Where both chronic tension and a loss of self-esteem have led to feelings of self-condemnation, it can assist in restoring to the Ethereal Soul an attitude of generosity and human kindness.

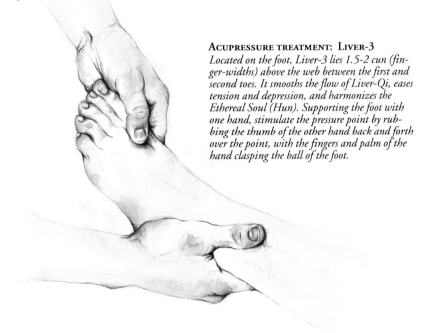

ACUPRESSURE TREATMENT: LIVER-3
Located on the foot, Liver-3 lies 1.5-2 cun (finger-widths) above the web between the first and second toes. It smooths the flow of Liver-Qi, eases tension and depression, and harmonizes the Ethereal Soul (Hun). Supporting the foot with one hand, stimulate the pressure point by rubbing the thumb of the other hand back and forth over the point, with the fingers and palm of the hand clasping the ball of the foot.

Depression of a Fire Nature

Depression of a Fire nature most often involves an imbalance of Joy and Love – the root emotions of the Heart and the Mind *(Shen)*. "Joy" is an extension of the *Shen's* innate sense of harmony and perfection, an experience of emotional and spiritual well-being. Love, too, is an expression of this aware-ness, of the way it is inspired by another.

The depression that afflicts the Heart and *Shen* involves a loss of *joie de vivre*, one's natural "joy of life". There is often a lack of enthusiasm and interest, and an inability to feel inspired. It tends to afflict those who are naturally warm and "emotional", but who, in disharmony, can become either cold and apathetic, or agitated and hypersensitive.

Due to the Fire Element's involvement with matters of love and friendship, Fire-type depression can also result from rejection. It is the anguish borne of emotional insecurity, and of disappointment in relationships. It is, in addition, a sad-ness of Spirit that can make one distant and unaffectionate, even when feelings of love are present.

Jasmine oil is a prime example of an aromatic for the depression of Fire. Its age-old reputation as an antidepressant and euphoric relates both to its warm, exotic, floral aroma and to its energetic action on the Heart. Here, its ability to gently tonify and, at the same time, relax the *Qi* of the Heart produces a comforting, uplifting effect on the emotions.

Associated with the Moon and the creative Feminine, jas-mine oil can reawaken a sense of warmth and aliveness in those who have grown cold and emotionally indifferent. It is also helpful for the depressive states that can originate from chronic sexual anxiety – whether the problem is one of in-hibition, self-restraint, frustration, or vulnerability.

Ylang ylang oil excels in this capacity, and enhances the expression of our delight in the sensuous. It is suitable for those whose need for emotional excitement can cause anxiety and depression when life seems dull. Helping us to fill our "emotional vacuum", it eases the despondency that comes of restless boredom.

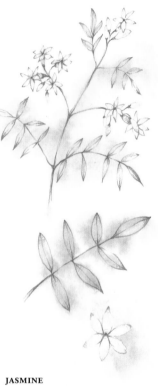

JASMINE

"Jasmine's cool, waxy flowers open to the sultry night air and must be picked before dawn to obtain the fragrance at its peak. They produce an essence infused with the sun's glory and the moon's magnetism."
Jane Grayson, *The Fragrant Year*

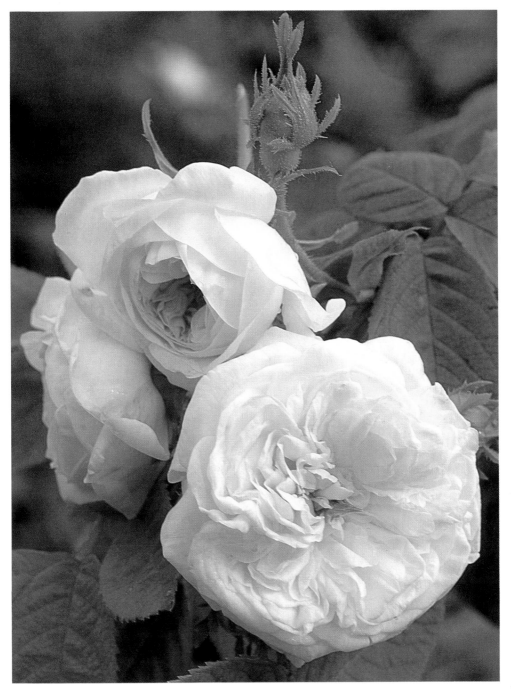

ROSE FLOWERS

The exquisitely soft and delicate petals of the rose flower – that wrap like sheaths around its cradled organs of reproduction – are like the layers of feeling that keep close to the heart. The tenderness of the flower is supported and protected by the adamant defences of its thorny branches. Though it nourishes the capacity for love, the oil protects our power to express it.

Rose oil is supportive of the Heart's *yin* energy, helping to restore a sense of emotional security. It is indicated for highly sensitive individuals who are quietly full of romantic idealism. Because they tend to expect so much from life and love, they are easily disappointed and hurt. Rose oil restores the capacity for self-fulfilment through helping to find the joy that lies within.

While jasmine and rose cool and calm the Heart, the uplifting effects of rosemary oil are due to its warming, invigorating nature. Indicated for a deficiency of the Heart's *yang* energy, it is appropriate for the sadness and apathy of those who suffer from physical and mental fatigue. Fortifying the Mind *(Shen)* and boosting the ego, it counteracts the depression that results from poor self-confidence, and from an inability to create goals that reveal one's true potential.

Melissa oil, also, is restorative to the Mind, and helps to disperse emotions that oppress and overwhelm. According to Nicholas Culpeper, melissa "reviveth the heart. . . and driveth away all troublesome cares and thoughts out of the mind, arising from melancholy and black choler". The term "black choler" points to heaviness or pessimism afflicting the *Shen's* natural state of harmony.

That the gentle "balm" is associated with the astrological sign of Cancer implies that the herb relates to problems that have their roots in childhood. We are clearly less able, during our early years, to resist oppressive emotional forces. The memory of being psychologically overpowered by others may continue to affect us as adults.

Melissa is suited, therefore, to emotionally delicate individuals who find it difficult to confront the causes of their depression. They "suffer in silence" rather than expose their discontent, and are reluctant to initiate change. Viewing the unknown with dread, they prefer to struggle with the known, however bleak and difficult.

Patchouli oil, through its earthy sweetness, is primarily associated with the Earth Element, yet can benefit depression of a Fire nature through inspiring an urge to explore and

Suggested Blends
(no. of drops per 20ml of /1tbsp of carrier)

COLD & JOYLESS
jasmine (3), ylang ylang (1), orange (1)

ABANDONED & BEREFT
rose (2), palmarosa (2), neroli (1)

DISPIRITED & DISHEARTENED
rosemary (4), ginger (1)

BLEAK WITH TEDIUM
coriander (3), patchouli (2), bergamot (1)

See Also
Coriander pp.64-5
Jasmine pp.84-5
Melissa pp.96-7
Patchouli pp.106-7
Rose pp.112-13
Rosemary pp.114-15
Ylang ylang pp.128-9

create. The oil may be used for depression in those who have lost their capacity for spontaneity and enjoyment, due to mental stress and strain.

Coriander seed oil, like patchouli, both comforts the Intellect *(Yi)* and uplifts the Mind *(Shen)*, benefiting those who are both worried and emotionally barren. It is helpful, in particular, for the depression that develops from a lack of variation and opportunity. Easing the oppression of the "daily grind", it instils an optimistic and inventive resourcefulness in those whose situation is one of repetitious duty.

ACUPRESSURE TREATMENT: HEART-5
Located on the front of the forearm, Heart-5 lies 1 cun (finger-width) directly above Heart-7, which is on the wrist crease, just inside the pisiform bone. Heart-5 reinforces the Qi of the Heart, and harmonizes and uplifts the Mind (Shen). Supporting the recipient's hand with one hand, stimulate the pressure point by rubbing the thumb of the other hand in a circular motion over the point, with the fingers and palm of the hand clasping the back of the forearm.

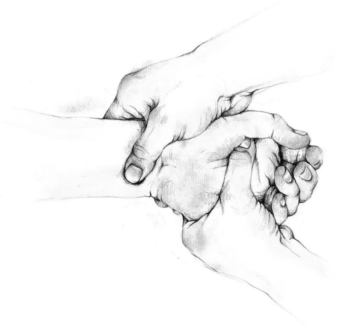

Depression of an Earth Nature

The type of depression that can be attributed to the Earth
Element involves, at one level, a disharmony of the Intellect
(Yi). When, due to a deficiency of the Spleen's *Qi-energy*, the
thinking process is strained and disrupted, the Intellect *(Yi)*
struggles for both clarity and calm, and becomes oppressed
by overthinking. The depressive feelings that develop are the
kind that are accompanied by worry and a sense of confusion. Fatigued and overburdened, the Intellect *(Yi)* is said to
suffer from an imbalance of Reflection – normally, a source
of quiet contemplation.

Reflection is one of the two root "emotions" that are associated with the Spleen and Earth Element. The other root
emotion is that of Sympathy – a term that reflects the caring,
nurturing aspect of Earth. Sympathy, here, is the psychological urge within us to support and serve, as well as our need to
feel supported. Belonging to the Element of practical
involvement, it is an emotion that tends to fulfil itself in
observable and consistent ways, in behaviour that we would
describe as "thoughtful".

An *excessive* degree of sympathy is evident in those who
constantly worry about, and show concern, for others. They
often neglect to see their *own* needs, and find it difficult to
admit to wanting help themselves.

There are, however, those in whom an overt need for
sympathy can produce a different type of imbalance. Rather
than displaying excessive self-sufficiency, such individuals are
prone to emotional dependency. Theirs is the depression of
unsatisfied emotional craving, and the embedded feeling that
"no one cares".

Whether the root problem involved is one of self-denial or
insecure neediness, the depressive state of the Earth Element
comes of a lack of self-nurturing, and the heaviness of Spirit
that follows.

The essential oils with sweet, predominantly base-note
fragrances tend to reinforce the Spleen and the Earth
Element. Their effects are generally stabilizing, nurturing,

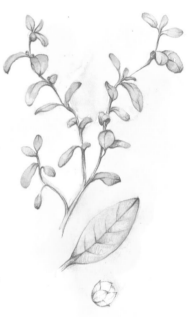

MARJORAM
*"Marjoram was considered sacred
to the Goddess Venus by the
Romans. It is still used in rituals in
her honour, and by those who
desire to find romantic fulfillment .
. . .Marjoram may be used in
either weddings or handfastings,
the custom from ancient Greece
calling for it to be woven into
wreaths to crown the newly
joined."*
Paul Beyerl, *The Master Book of
Herbalism*

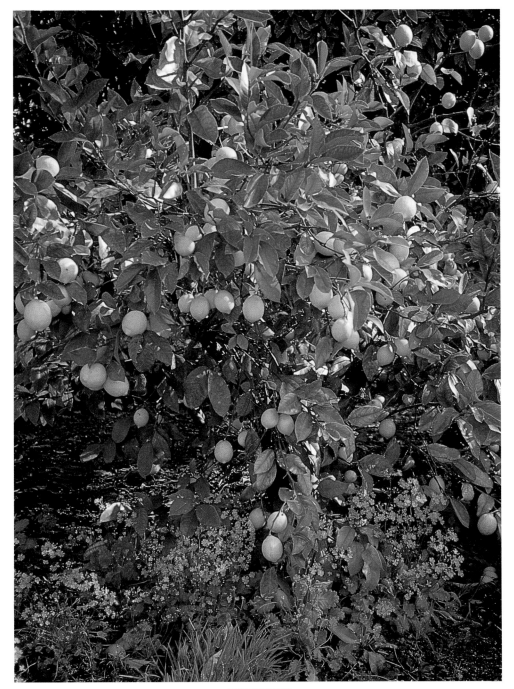

LEMON TREES

*"Spiritually-physically [lemon oil] has a cooling and clearing, bright
and refreshing effect. It has a strong relationship with light through
its cultivation regions and through the colour of the fruit ... The oil is
recommended to be used where there is an inner conflict between
mental affinity and conscious attitude, in order to come to a clear,
consciously settled solution."* Dietrich Gumbel, *Principles of
Holistic Skin Therapy with Herbal Essences*

and desensitizing. One of the most uplifting of these is
vetiver oil.

The power of vetiver oil to nurture and promote absorption benefits, on a subtle level, a propensity toward
self-denial. Its rich, resinous nature conveys an experience of
sustenance, and helps to reconnect us to the body. It is indicated, in particular, for the type of depression suffered by
those who habitually neglect their needs. They drive themselves hard, and may take little time out for food and rest,
hiding beneath a capable exterior a diminished sense of
emotional self-worth.

Marjoram is another oil that has the power to comfort and
nurture, and soothes a heavy Spirit devoid of calm contentment. It is associated through it sweetness, and its ability to
promote digestion, mainly with the Earth Element.
However, as a respiratory tonic and Funeral Herb on the one
hand, and as a Herb of Love on the other, the oil can be
linked, in addition, to the Metal and Fire Elements.
Marjoram may be used, therefore, for the sadness of loss and
the gloom of isolation. In either case, the despondency
involved is characterized by a craving to give and receive –
to nurture and be nurtured.

Cardamom oil may also be associated with Earth, and can
be recommended for the despondency of indifference.
Stimulating the Intellect *(Yi)* and an "appetite for life", it
helps to uplift the person who complains of apathy and lack
of interest – particularly when they are burdened with
responsibilities.

Lemon oil clarifies the Intellect *(Yi)*, and lightens the Spirit
through its ability to refresh. When the mind becomes "congested" with negative thoughts and worries, the oil will help
to unburden, and to restore a sense of light-hearted ease. Its
ability to clear and illuminate the mind make it appropriate
for the sense of oppression that comes of being mentally
"bogged down" and disorientated.

Frankincense and myrrh oils not only clarify and still the
mind but also awaken and expand one's spiritual consciousness.

Suggested Blends

*(no. of drops per 20ml/1tbsp
of carrier)*

DEPRESSIVE SELF-NEGLECT
vetiver (3), cardamom (1), rose (1)
LONELY & FORLORN
*marjoram (3), rosemary (2),
myrrh (1)*
BURDENED & HUMOURLESS
lemon (3), jasmine (2)
OPPRESSIVE OVER-ATTACHMENT
*frankincense (2), myrrh (2),
cypress (2)*

See Also

Cardamom pp.56-7
Frankincense pp.74-5
Lemon pp.92-3
Marjoram pp.94-5
Myrrh pp.98-9
Vetiver pp.124-5

Their serenely resinous fragrances imbue a profound sense of tranquillity, comparable only to that of sandalwood and spikenard. Frankincense oil alleviates the overthinking that overwhelms the Intellect and constricts the Bodily Soul. It is helpful for the depression of those who feel burdened with concerns of an intractable or mundane nature. It encourages insight, detachment, and transcendence, and the spiritual strength to endure and relinquish.

Myrrh oil, too, helps to free us from the oppression of worldly limitation and misfortune. Soothing the pain that weighs down the Self, it helps us to access our spiritual will – our capacity for self-discipline and transformative awareness.

Both frankincense and myrrh are traditional Funeral Herbs, and help us to grieve and come to terms with the past. They may be associated, from this perspective, with the Metal Element. Myrrh, in particular, works to comfort the sorrow of loss, and allows us to see through the eye of eternity.

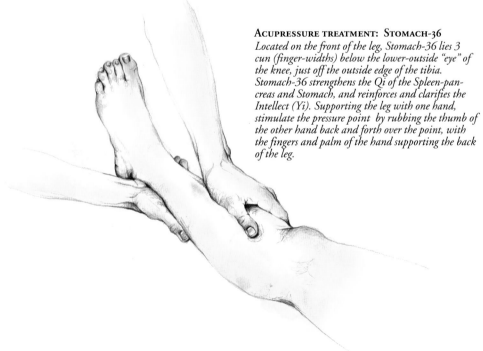

ACUPRESSURE TREATMENT: STOMACH-36
Located on the front of the leg, Stomach-36 lies 3 cun (finger-widths) below the lower-outside "eye" of the knee, just off the outside edge of the tibia. Stomach-36 strengthens the Qi of the Spleen-pancreas and Stomach, and reinforces and clarifies the Intellect (Yi). Supporting the leg with one hand, stimulate the pressure point by rubbing the thumb of the other hand back and forth over the point, with the fingers and palm of the hand supporting the back of the leg.

Depression of a Metal Nature

The Metal Element incorporates that part of our being we often call the "vital body". The Bodily Soul *(P'o)*, is housed by the Lungs, and lives through the experience of the senses. It provides an instinctive and vibrant sense of aliveness, living fully in the moment when unhindered and strong. The type of negative emotions that afflict the Bodily Soul are those that impede its vitality and presence, and its power to accept and relinquish. Feelings of pessimism, regret, and remorse, and of experiences of loss that we have failed to come to terms with, all constrict the Bodily Soul and result in a disharmony of Metal.

The root emotion of the Lungs and of the Metal Element generally is that of Grief. Like Fear and Anger, Grief has an important and positive role to play, as the process of both accepting and of letting go of loss. It only becomes a disharmonious emotion when the process is impaired and loss is made unconscious or vaguely pervasive.

The depression of a Metal nature often involves, therefore, an experience of grief that one has never come to terms with. Because there is an inability truly to grieve or weep, the individual is oppressed instead by a feeling of emotional vacancy. A sense of melancholy, remoteness, and resignation predominate, reflecting a wound as yet too deep to heal.

One of the most clearly indicated oils for this type of depression is cypress. Like frankincense and myrrh, it was traditionally employed as a Funeral Herb, and, through providing a source of spiritual comfort, was thought to be of value in the grieving process. Its energetic action to both *contain* and *move* the *blood* reflects its ability, on a subtle level, to facilitate change and transition generally. Represented by Pluto – a symbol of transformation – it encourages us to relinquish that which no longer serves or fulfils us.

It is therefore indicated for the depression of the individual who is in some way "stuck" and unable to move forward. Whether they persistently feel submerged by a profound sense of loss, or are oppressed by circumstances they dare not

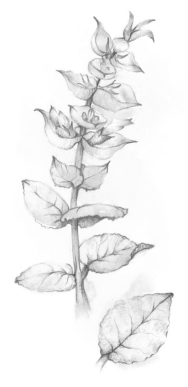

CLARY SAGE
"Sclary, as the herbalists say, is good for the hot gout. Sclary clarifieth her voice that hath been hoarse, and she is right good both to the lungs, and to the gullet and the bowel, and many virtues she hath, of which the wise women train."
Macer's Herbal, 12th century

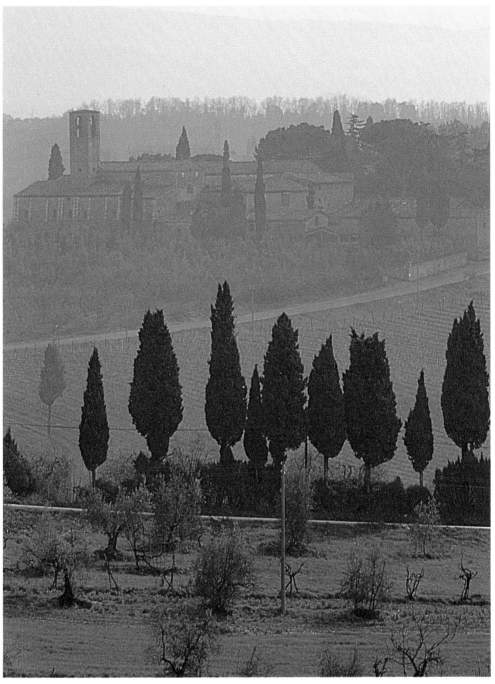

CYPRESS TREES
"Sweeter than the finest nectar
Of the honeyed pomegranate
Is the fragrance of the wind
In the grove of cypress."
The Essene Gospel of Peace, Book Two
(trans. Edmond Bordeaux Szekely)

change, their depressive feelings are characterized by a feeling of mournful stasis.

Eucalyptus oil is also helpful for an inability to move forward, and benefits depressive states of "spiritual contraction". It "opens the chest" and encourages a more expansive sense of awareness, invigorating the Bodily Soul and sharpening the senses. It may be used to uplift the Spirit when there is feeling of entrapment and limitation – when the person in question yearns for greater "freedom of Spirit".

Clary sage oil is renowned for its antidepressant properties, and concentrates its action on both the Bodily Soul and Intellect. It is perhaps the classic essential oil for melancholy, and for a feeling of restless distraction, fortifying the "vital spirits" and smoothing the flow of *Qi*.

It is suited, in particular, for the type of depression that accrues from chronic tension and nervous strain. As clary sage oil both relaxes and reinforces the nervous system, it restores a feeling of inner strength when we have overstretched ourselves.

From a more subtle perspective, clary sage oil may be used to uplift the Spirit where oppressive feelings of confusion have mounted. Like Roman and German chamomile, it eases the tension that results from contradictory tendencies and desires. Clarifying and reviving our instinctive sense of knowing, it disperses the clouds that gather over states of inner conflict.

Hyssop and pine oils, like cypress and eucalyptus, encourage us to outgrow the limited and to "let go" of the outworn. Although not as deeply transforming as cypress oil for embedded feelings of loss, pine, in particular, helps to ease regret, and to dissipate remorse. Where both hyssop and pine oil excel, however, is for feelings of "negativity".

When the Bodily Soul is flourishing, and vitality is good, there is a general sense of optimism, and a capacity for openness. When depleted and constricted, however, the Bodily Soul is vulnerable, and easily succumbs to outside pressures that can undermine or demoralize. Strong, fresh and

Suggested Blends
(no. of drops per 20ml / 1 tbsp of carrier)

Persistent sense of loss
cypress (4), frankincense (1), rose (1)

Melancholic & distant
clary sage (3), rosemary (2), thyme (1)

Wretched & remorseful
pine (3), marjoram (2), cypress (1)

Negative & pessimistic
hyssop (2), clary sage (2), orange (2)

See Also
Clary sage pp.62-3
Cypress pp.66-7
Eucalyptus pp.68-9
Hyssop pp.82-3
Pine pp.110-11
Tea tree pp.120-1

exhilarating, hyssop and pine oils help to abate such vulnerability, and disperse the pessimism of a jaded outlook. They are useful for the negative attitude that can so often accompany fatigue and exhaustion.

Tea tree, finally, is another protective oil – a major tonic of the body's *Defensive-Qi*. Lending strength to both the Bodily Soul *(P'o)* and Mind *(Shen)*, it helps to boost the morale of those whose health is poor. When combined with oils appropriate for the individual, it is especially useful for depression in the person whose immune system is weak.

ACUPRESSURE TREATMENT: LUNG-7
Located on the front of the forearm, Lung-7 lies over the radial artery, 1.5 cun (finger-widths) above the wrist crease. Lung-7 activates the movement of Lung-Qi, and revitalizes and uplifts the Bodily Soul (P'o). Supporting the recipient's hand with one hand, stimulate the pressure point by rubbing the thumb of the other hand back and forth over the point, with the fingers and palm of the hand clasping the back of the forearm.

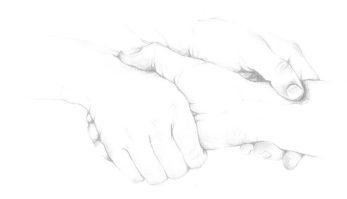

Depression of a Water Nature

The type of depression that is associated with the Water Element is centred around an imbalance of the Will (Zhi). The Will, in harmony, is a source of initiative and will-power, and makes an important contribution to our confidence and stamina. It is stored in the Kidney, which – the root of yin and yang – affords us our basic, constitutional strength.

The depressive state of a Water nature can involve, therefore, a feeling of powerlessness or apathy. Individuals in question may feel, for example, when faced with difficult circumstances, suddenly overwhelmed by forces beyond their control. They doubt their capacity to cope with challenging situations, and are plunged into a state of despair when life seems to demand too much of them. The demoralized feelings that "crush" the Spirit are often intermingled with a sense of fear.

A different kind of negative outlook may involve, in contrast, no known cause – though it may have its roots in childhood. Here, the Will is stricken for no apparent reason, and in those who are free from oppressive problems. The depression that results may be described as "existential", and reflect, to some extent, a loss of will to live.

Whether the cause is known or unkown, thyme essential oil helps to counteract depression in all those situations that require a buttressing of the Will. Like rosemary and tea tree oils, it is a powerful neurotonic, celebrated for centuries as a source of bravery. With an equally potent action on the Bodily Soul (P'o) of the Lungs, it instils in those who are discouraged and dejected a vibrant and determined optimism. Thyme oil is indicated, therefore, for depressive states of defeat or dread, as well as those of apathy.

Juniper berry oil is similar in influence, and reinforces, like thyme, both the Will and Bodily Soul. It is helpful, in particular, for the depressive states of those who, due to deep self-doubt and disinterest, "give-up" within and avoid all challenges. When burdened with responsibilities they cannot

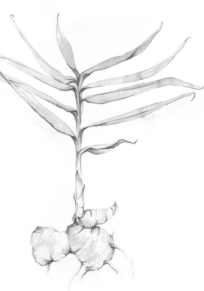

GINGER
"Ginger is perhaps the best and most sattvic [pure and subtle] of spices. It was called vishwabhesaj, the 'universal medicine'. Dry ginger is drier and hotter than fresh. It is a better stimulant and expectorant for reducing Kapha [mucus] and increasing Agni [vital fire]. Fresh ginger is a better diaphoretic, better for colds, coughs, vomiting and for deranged Vata [vital energy]."
Dr Vasant Lad and David Frawley, The Yoga of Herbs

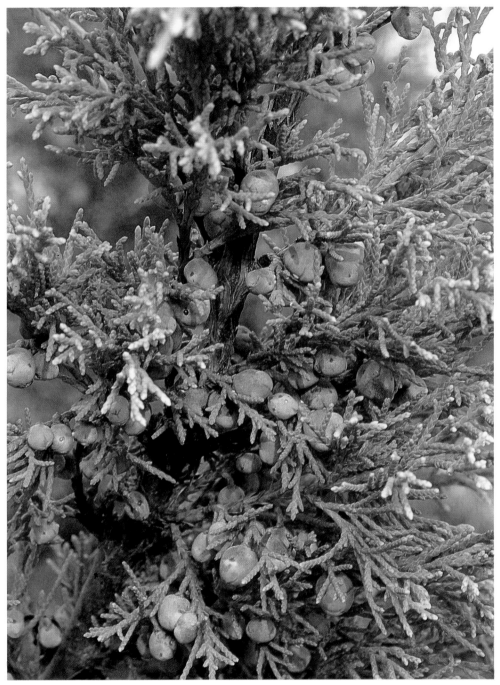

JUNIPER BERRIES
*The juniper bush is unique in being both hardy and independent,
favouring the type of barren heathland that other shrubs avoid. Its prickly
branches and the bitterness of the berries help it to retain its fruits for as
long as three years at a time. The oil that it yields conveys fortitude and
resolve, and is suited to those who tackle life alone.*

avoid, they tend to isolate themselves and worry – rather than taking affirmative action. Juniper berry oil is suited to those who have let negativity make them fixed and rigid in outlook, and who have allowed a fear of failure to block their efforts at progress.

Cypress oil, too, helps us to move forward psychologically, and is in this sense important for a depression of a Metal nature. Its profound action on the Will *(Zhi)* makes it relevant, in addition, for the type of depression associated with the Water Element. Helping us to access the fears and anxieties that we have pushed below the reach of consciousness, it is appropriate for those depressive states that seem to lack a specific origin.

Cypress oil, in addition, is indicated for the person who links their depression with the feeling of being controlled and manipulated. Because their Will is stricken or submerged, it is easily overpowered by the Will of others, and results in a feeling of oppression.

Ginger oil, like thyme, will help an apathetic type of depression, and, combined with other essences, uplifts the Mind *(Shen)*. Warming the *yang* and energizing the Will, it boosts morale and sparks initiative. It disperses the gloom of those who are submerged by a sense of inertia, and helps us respond to depressive states that call for confident and self-assured action.

The final type of depression of a Water nature is helped by geranium oil. While ginger ignites the Will, and spurs us on to action, geranium cools, settles and restrains it, encouraging us to relax and renew our resources. It is therefore suitable for depressive states that result from overwork, and for the depletion of those who have driven themselves to the limit. While clary sage oil is also indicated for the effects of "nervous burn-out", it is more appropriate for people with stagnant *Qi-energy*. Geranium oil, in contrast, is best employed for those whose condition is *hot* in nature and deficient in *yin*.

Suggested Blends
(no. of drops per 20ml/1tbsp of carrier)

Discouraged and dejected
thyme (2), rosemary (2)

Oppressed by others
cypress (3), juniper (2)

Deep inertia of the spirit
cypress (4), ginger (2)

Driven to nervous exhaustion
geranium (2), sandalwood (2), jasmine (1)

See Also
Cypress pp.66-7
Geranium pp.76-7
Ginger pp.78-9
Juniper pp.86-7
Thyme pp.122-3

It should again be kept in mind – as in the case of any disharmony – that the depressive state of the person may reflect an
imbalance in more than one Element.

For example, if the moody irritability of the Wood-type
depression combines with the loss of *joie de vivre* found with
a disharmony of Fire, chamomile and jasmine oils may be
blended together. Similarly, if the mentally burdened and
worrisome depression of Earth is coupled with the remorse
and pessimism of Metal, one may blend frankincense oil
with pine.

ACUPRESSURE TREATMENT: KIDNEY-6
*Located on the inside of the ankle, Kidney-6 lies 1 cun (fin-
ger-width) directly below the medial malleolus (ankle bone).
Kidney-6 supports the yin, calms the Mind and "opens the
chest", helping to alleviate both anxiety and depression of a
Water nature. Supporting the heel with one hand, stimulate
the pressure point by rubbing the thumb in a circular motion
over the point.*

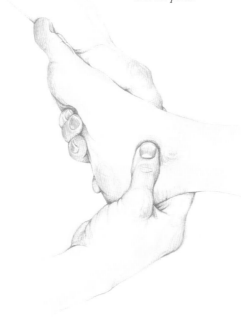

Problems in Relating

oils for love and friendship

There are many commonly used essential oils that are of potential benefit for problems in relating, although those surveyed here may be considered the most important. While an emphasis will be placed on relationships of a sexual and romantic nature, these essential oils can pertain equally to relating as a whole.

All Five Elements play a role in human relationships – in ways that vary according to the individual. However, the Element that predominates in all relationships is the one that constitutes our emotional core – the Fire Element. Home of the Heart and Mind *(Shen)*, it is the principal source of sensitive awareness, and of the root emotions of Joy and Love.

One of the most renowned of aromatics for enhancing joy and love is jasmine oil. Traditionally considered a Fertility Herb, jasmine is a potent aphrodisiac. It is indicated, in particular, for the habitually self-restrained and emotionally inhibited individual. Though ideally they would wish to express warmth freely, they find it difficult to do so due to vulnerability and a lack of confidence.

The action of ylang ylang oil is similar in nature – though with a greater emphasis on easing *sexual* anxiety. With its aphrodisiac and euphoric properties closely intertwined, its flowers are strewn on the beds of Indonesian newlyweds.

Patchouli oil is another sexual tonic that originates from Southeast Asia. It may be used by those whose work involves a high degree of pressure and mental strain. In intimate moments they find it difficult to relax and to fully inhabit their sensuality. The musky, earthy scent of patchouli oil can facilitate love-making through lulling the mind and warming the body.

Cardamom oil – like patchouli, more Earth than Fire – also enhances a desire for intimacy. It is suited to those who, though glad to feel needed, are afraid of being "absorbed", and of losing their self-identity.

Ginger oil, too, is a sexual tonic – yet entirely different to, say, jasmine or ylang ylang. While these sweet, floral essences encourage us to relax, ginger is spicy, *hot*, and invigorating. It

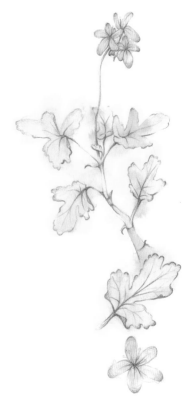

GERANIUM
The only region where geranium grows wild is in the Cape Province of South Africa. In this one area of the world, over 600 species of Pelargonium flourish. It prefers light, well-drained soils that retain little moisture – producing one of the best essential oils for dry conditions of the skin. The oil, in addition, restores the "moistness" of sensitivity.

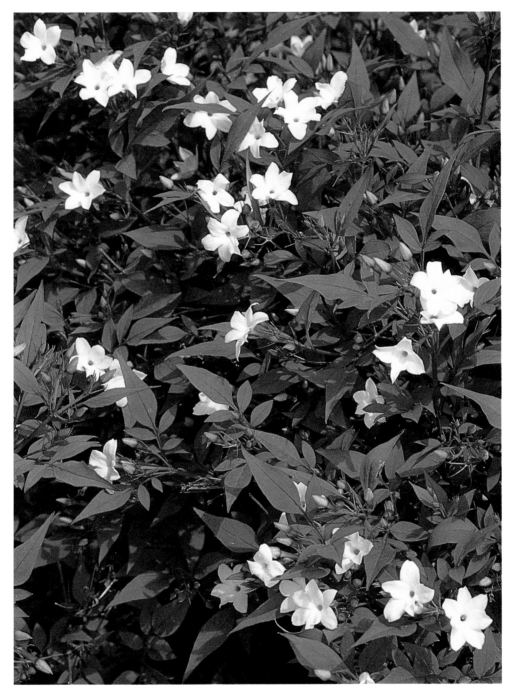

JASMINE FLOWERS

*In China, where jasmine flower is a symbol of womanly sweetness,
it was a traditional custom for women to decorate their hair with
the buds. After dark, the buds would begin to open, becoming more
heavenly scented as the night wore on, their perfume accentuated
by the warmth of the body.*

will help to exhilarate the type of cold and debilitated individual who, due to deficient *Kidney-yang,* lacks sexual vitality.

Juniper berry oil also warms the Kidneys, promoting both vigor and self-assurance. Although it is not a sexual tonic, it benefits those, who due to worry and self-absorption, cut themselves off emotionally. It may be combined with fennel essential oil to encourage confident self-expression.

While ginger and juniper oils invigorate the *yang,* and support our extrovert nature, geranium and sandalwood strengthen the *yin* energy of the body/mind, and enhance receptivity. Geranium oil is appropriate for those who are eager to please, but who, due to underlying insecurity, make it difficult for others to give to *them.*

While those in need of geranium are often divorced from their feelings, the individual helped by lavender oil tends to be emotionally oversensitive – and can be shy and self-conscious as a result. Melissa oil, too, will calm the delicate and susceptible – the person who cannot bear the thought of confrontation and conflict. Gently helping them to stand their ground, the oil supports those who are easily dominated. Clarifying the Mind *(Shen)* and dispersing oppressive feelings, melissa oil, in addition, is helpful for suspicion and distrust. It shares with lemon oil a capacity to "open the heart" – yet with a clarity free of *naiveté.*

It is this very combination of wisdom and loving trust that essential oil of rose seeks ultimately to "teach" – the consummate Herb of Love. It helps to heal those who are too insecure to fully trust another, due to past experiences of rejection and emotional wounding. Rose may be used, therefore, like palmarosa oil, for feelings of possessiveness and jealousy. It will, on the other hand, help to cure emotional coldness, healing the scars of love's sharp thorns.

While rose soothes the pain that results in insecurity, neroli oil eases the kind that is revealed through self-denial. The "neroli-type" of individual *represses* their emotional wounds, and subsequently displays deep conflicts of charac-

Suggested Blends
(no. of drops per 20ml/1tbsp of carrier)

SEXUALLY INHIBITED
jasmine (3), ylang ylang (1), sandalwood (1)

INSECURE & UNYIELDING
geranium (2), patchouli (2), bergamot (2)

VULNERABLE & UNTRUSTING
rose (2), palmarosa (2), lemon (1)

FEAR OF COMMITMENT
caraway (2), cardamom (2), rose (1)

See Also

ter. They may, for example, engage in sexual relationships that leave them emotionally dissatisfied and cold – or, instead, cling to those, that while stable and supportive, possess little passion or joy.

Two final oils for problems in relating are supportive in particular to the Earth Element. Caraway oil – a traditional symbol of constancy – helps to foster the strength of commitment. With a parallel action on the Will *(Zhi)* of the Kidneys, it placates the fear of emotional entrapment. Marjoram oil, in contrast, is reassuring and comforting, and eases feelings of emotional deprivation. Soothing the pain of loneliness, it promotes, in a similar way to, rose oil, the ability to nurture oneself.

ACUPRESSURE TREATMENT: PERICARDIUM-7

Located on the front of the wrist, Pericardium-7 lies on the mid-point of the wrist crease. Pericardium-7 settles the Qi of the Heart, and calms and comforts the Mind (Shen). It is particularly indicated for emotional problems within relationships. Supporting the recipient's hand with one hand, stimulate the pressure point by rubbing the thumb of the other hand in a circular motion over the point, with the fingers and palm of the hand clasping the back of the wrist. Stimulating Heart-7 will support the action of Pericardium-7.

Main Chemical Constituents

BENZOIN esters incl. coniferyl benzoate; acids incl. benzoic & cinnamic acid

BERGAMOT esters incl. linalyl acetate; terpenes incl. limonene; alcohols incl. linalol; furocoumarins incl. bergaptene

CARAWAY ketones incl. carvone; terpenes incl. limonene & carvene

CARDAMOM oxides incl. cineole; esters incl. terpinyl acetate; alcohols incl. linalol

CEDARWOOD (Cedrus atlantica) terpenes incl. cedrene; alcohols incl. atlantol; ketones incl. atlantone

CHAMOMILE Chamaemeleum nobile: esters incl. isobutyl angelate; ketones incl. pinocarvone; Chamomilla recutita: oxides incl. bisabolol oxide; alcohols incl. bisabolol; terpenes incl. farnesene & chamazulene

CLARY SAGE esters incl. linalyl acetate; alcohols incl. linalol & sclareol; terpenes incl. germacrene

CORIANDER alcohols incl. linalol & thymol; esters incl. linalyl acetate; terpenes incl. caryophyllene

CYPRESS terpenes incl. pinene; alcohols incl. cedrol; aldehydes incl. terpinyl acetate

EUCALYPTUS (Eucalyptus globulus) oxides incl. cineole; terpenes incl. pinene; alcohols incl. globulol

EVERLASTING esters incl. neryl acetate; diones incl. italidiones

FENNEL methyl-ether phenols incl. anethole; terpenes incl. limonene; alcohols incl. fenchol; ketones incl. fenchone

FRANKINCENSE terpenes incl. pinene, cymene & limonene; alcohols incl. borneol

GERANIUM alcohols incl. citronellol, geraniol & linalol; esters incl. citronellyl formates; aldehydes incl. geranial

GINGER terpenes incl. zingiberine, phellandrene & curcumene; alcohols incl. citronellol & linalol

GRAPEFRUIT terpenes incl. limonene; ketones incl. nooketone; aldehydes incl. citral; furocoumarins incl. bergaptole

HYSSOP ketones incl. pinocamphone; terpenes incl. pinene; methyl-ether phenols incl. myrtenyl methyl ether

JASMINE aldehydes incl. benzyl acetate; alcohols incl. phytol, linalol, jasmone & eugenol

JUNIPER terpenes incl. pinene, sabinene, limonene & germacrene; alcohols incl. terpineol

LAUREL oxides incl. cineole; terpenes incl. pinene; alcohols incl. linalol

LAVENDER (Lavandula angustifolia) esters incl. linalyl acetate & lavandulyl acetate; alcohols incl. linalol & terpineol

LEMON terpenes incl. limonene; aldehydes incl. geranial; furocoumarins incl. bergaptole

MARJORAM (Origanum marjorana) alcohols incl. terpineol, thujanol & linalol; terpenes incl. terpinene

MELISSA aldehydes incl. geranial, neral & citronellal; terpenes incl. caryophyllene & germacrene

MYRRH terpenes incl. elemene & copaene; ketones incl. methylisobutyl ketone

NEROLI alcohols incl. linalol & terpineol; terpenes incl. pinene & limonene; esters incl linalyl acetate

ORANGE terpenes incl. limonene; alcohols incl. linalol; ketones incl carvone

PALMAROSA alcohols incl. geraniol & linalol; esters incl. geranyl acetate; terpenes incl. limonene

PATCHOULI alcohols incl. patchouolol; terpenes incl. bulnesene; oxides incl. bulnesene oxide

PEPPERMINT alcohols incl. menthol; ketones incl. menthone & piperitone; oxides incl. cineole

PINE (Pinus sylvestris) terpenes incl. pinene & limonene; esters incl. bornyl acetate; alcohols incl. borneol

ROSE alcohols incl. citronellol & geraniol; terpenes incl. stearoptene

ROSEMARY oxides incl. cineole; terpenes incl. pinene & camphene; ketones incl. camphor; alcohols incl. borneol

SANDALWOOD alcohols incl. santalol; terpenes incl. santalene

SPIKENARD terpenes incl. patchoulene & gurjunene; ketones incl. aristolenone; alcohols incl. patchouli alcohol

TEA TREE alcohols incl. terpineol; terpenes incl. terpinene; oxides incl. cineole

THYME (Thymus vulgaris thymoliferum) phenols incl. thymol & carvacrol; terpenes incl. cymene; alcohols incl. linalol

VETIVER alcohols incl. vetiverol; ketones incl. vetivone; esters incl. vetiverol acetate

YARROW terpenes incl. sabinene, chamazulene & germacrene; alcohols incl. borneol; oxides incl. cineole; ketones incl. camphor

YLANG YLANG alcohols incl. linalol; terpenes incl. germacrene; esters incl. geranyl acetate; methyl ether phenols incl. cresol methyl ether

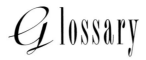 lossary

Anticoagulant – inhibits the coagulation of blood

Antihaematomic – disperses the accumulation of clotted blood

Antineuralgic – relieves nerve pain

Antisudorific – restrains perspiration

Antisclerotic – prevents the hardening of tissue

Antiseborrhoeic – restrains the production of sebum, the oily substance secreted by the sweat glands

Aperient – mildly laxative

Astringent – causes contraction of living tissues, esp. of mucous membranes

Balsamic – soothing; with the quality of a balsam

Calmative – relaxing

Cardiotonic – strengthens the heart

Carminative – relieves flatulence

Cephalic – benefits the head and brain

Cholagogue – promotes bile flow through stimulating the gall bladder

Choleretic – promotes the secretion of bile by the liver

Depurative – removes impurities from the blood; detoxifying

Diaphoretic – promotes perspiration

Diuretic – increases urination

Dysmenorrhoea – menstrual pain

Emmenagogue – promotes menstruation

Emollient – soothes the skin

Epigastrium – the stomach region

Expectorant – promotes the expulsion of mucous

Febrifuge – reduces fever

Hermidical – fights infection

Haemostatic – arrests bleeding

Hepatic – relating to, or benefiting, the liver

Hypertensive – counteracts low blood pressure

Hypotensive – counteracts high blood pressure

Ischaemic – involving a reduction in blood supply

Lactogenic – promotes the secretion of milk

Leucorrhoea – vaginal discharge

Lipolytic – breaks down fat

Litholytic – breaks down stones

Menorrhagia – excessive menstrual bleeding

Neurotonic – strengthens the nervous system

Ophthalmic – relating to, and benefiting, the eyes

Otitis – inflammation of the ear

Parturient – aids childbirth

Peristalsis – an involuntary muscular wave-like movement of the alimentary canal

Phlebotonic – strengthens the veins

Phototoxicity – a substance that can increase, to the point of toxicity, the sensitivity of the skin to sunlight, and to ultraviolet radiation generally

Prostatic – relating to the prostate gland

Rubefacient – increases local blood circulation, causing redness of the skin

Sialogogue – stimulates the secretion of saliva

Stomachic – promotes stomach function

Sudorific – promotes sweating

Tachycardia – an abnormally rapid heart rate

Terrain – underlying energetic condition

Tonic – strengthening

Unguent – ointment

Uterine – relating to, and benefiting, the uterus

Vasoconstrictor – causes narrowing of the blood vessels

Vasodilator – causes dilation of the blood vessels

Vermifuge – expels intestinal worms

Vulnerary – promotes the healing of wounds

Further Reading & Addresses

Books

The Master Book of Herbalism, Beyerl, P., Phoenix Publishing Inc., 1984

Between Heaven and Earth: A Guide to Chinese Medicine, Beinfield, H. & Korngold, E., Ballantine Books, 1992

Aromatherapy A-Z, Davis, P., Beekman, 1991

Kitchen Pharmacy, Elliot, R. & De Paoli, C., Morrow, 1993

The Energetics of Western Herbs, Vols I & II, Holmes, P., Artemis Press, 1989

Aromatherapy: A Complete Guide to the Healing Art, Green, M., Crossing Press, 1995

Shiatsu: The Complete Guide, Jarmey, C. & Mojay, G, Thorsons, 1991

The Complete Woman's Herbal, McIntyre, A., Henry Holt, 1994

Aromatherapy for Common Ailments, Price, S., Simon and Schuster, 1990

Aromatherapy: The Encyclopedia of Plants and Oils and How They Help You, Ryman, D., Bantam, 1993

Aromatherapy Handbook, Ryman, D., Atrium, 1995

Author's acknowledgments
I am deeply indebted to my friend, Carlo De Paoli, for his insight and inspiration. I would like to thank Ruth Smith, the Institute's senior massage tutor, and Alex Brooke, her assistant, for their invaluable help in the preparation of the massage illustrations. My thanks goes, too, to Jan Kusmirek for his revealing thoughts on essential oils, and to Anne Neele for her help in preparing material for Part I of the book. I am grateful to Susan Mears, my literary agent, for her hard work and enthusiasm, and to Joanna Godfrey Wood, my editor, for her patient commitment and keen judgment. And finally, I would like to thank Carol-Ann Honyben for her general advice, and for her assistance in researching the botanical aspects of the plants.

Photographic credits
Phil Gamble p.2; The Garden Picture Library p.135 p.147, p.151, p.167 p.179 (John Glover); p.139 (Mayer/Le Scanff); p.155 (Laslo Puskas); p.159 (Linda Burgess); p.171 (Gary Rogers); p.183 (Clive Boursnell); Images p.8, p.49, p.130, p.175; Gabriel Mojay p.143

Useful addresses

The Institute of Traditional Herbal Medicine and Aromatherapy
P.O. Box 6555, London N8 9DF, UK
Tel: (01144) 181-348-3755 (for details of seminars and courses in USA, with Gabriel Mojay)

The American Alliance of Aromatherapy
Melissa Jochim, P.O. Box 309, Depoe Bay, Or. 97341
Tel: 800-809-9850 (for registered therapists)

The National Association for Holistic Aromatherapy
National Office: P.O. Box 17622, Boulder, Co. 80308
Tel: 800-566-6735 (for registered therapists)

The Aromatherapy Guide
Susan Hollick, Vencom Publishing Inc., 24 Hanover Road, Suite 2205, Brampton, Ontario L6S 5K8, Canada
Tel: 908-799-2108 (annual publication of information relevant to USA and Canada)

Publisher's acknowledgments
Gaia Books would like to thank the following for their help in the production of this book:
Hazel Bell (index), Jan Dunkley, Lesley Gilbert, Cathy Meeus, Hannah Wheeler and Linley Joy Clode.

Illustration credits
Illustrations on these pages first appeared in *Symbols, Signs and Signets* by Ernst Lehner and are reproduced here with kind permission of Constable and Co. Ltd: pp.10, 12, 51, 55, 57, 59, 61, 63, 65, 67, 71, 73, 75, 77, 79, 81, 83, 85, 87, 89, 91, 93, 95, 97, 99, 101, 103, 109, 111, 113, 115, 117, 119, 123, 125, 127. Those on pp.53, 69, 121 first appeared in *The Encyclopedia of Signs and Symbols* by John Laing and David Wire and are reproduced here with the kind permission of Studio Editions. Those on pp. 105, 107, 129 first appeared in *Sexual Secrets* by Nik Douglas and Penny Slinger and are reproduced here with the kind permission of Destiny Books. The illustration on p. 47 first appeared in *The Book of Signs* by Rudolf Koch and is reproduced here with the kind permission of Dover Publications.

Index

Main subject references are **bold**;
illustration and caption references are *italic*.